also by David Wilson

BODY AND ANTIBODY: A REPORT ON THE NEW IMMUNOLOGY (1972)

THE NEW ARCHAEOLOGY (1975)

THESE ARE BORZOI BOOKS, PUBLISHED IN NEW YORK BY ALFRED A. KNOPF

In Search of
PENICILLIN

In Search of
PENICILLIN

David Wilson

 ALFRED A. KNOPF, New York, 1976

THIS IS A BORZOI BOOK
PUBLISHED BY ALFRED A. KNOPF, INC.

Copyright © 1976 by David Wilson
All rights reserved under International and Pan-American Copyright
Conventions. Published in the United States by Alfred A. Knopf, Inc.,
New York, and simultaneously in Canada by Random House of Canada
Limited, Toronto. Distributed by Random House, Inc., New York.
Published in Great Britain by Faber and Faber Limited, London.

LIBRARY OF CONGRESS CATALOGING IN PUBLICATION DATA
Wilson, David, [Date] In search of penicillin.
Bibliography: p.
Includes index.
1. Penicillin—History. I. Title. [DNLM 1. Penicillin—History. QV354 W747p]
RS165.P38W54 1976   615'.329'23   75-36806
ISBN 0-394-40108-5

Manufactured in the United States of America

First Edition

To Andrew

CONTENTS

ACKNOWLEDGMENTS

I am grateful to the Royal Society for permission to quote extracts from a lecture, "Thirty Years of Penicillin Therapy," by Professor Sir Ernst Boris Chain, published as *Proc. Roy. Soc.* (1971) B.179, pp. 293–319.

Other sources I wish to acknowledge are *The Birth of Penicillin* by Ronald Hare (George Allen & Unwin, 1970); *The Life of Sir Alexander Fleming* by André Maurois (Jonathan Cape, 1959); *Rise Up to Life* by Lennard Bickel (Angus & Robertson, 1972); *Miracle Drug* by David Masters (Eyre and Spottiswoode, 1946); *The Doctor's Dilemma* by George Bernard Shaw (Constable, 1930); *Penicillin* by Boris Sokoloff (George Allen & Unwin, 1946); *Fleming, Discoverer of Penicillin* by L.J. Ludovici (Andrew Dakers, 1952); *The Life Savers* by Ritchie Calder (Pan Books, 1961); and *The Penicillin Group of Drugs* by G.T. Stewart (Elsevier, 1965).

Short quotations have been taken from the following academic publications (details are contained in the references at the end of the book): *British Journal of Experimental Pathology; Lancet; Royal Society of Public Health & Hygiene Journal; Kungl Boktrichereit,* P.A., Stockholm (Norstedt & Soner, 1947); *Proceedings of the Royal Society,* and *Biographical Memoirs of Fellows of the Royal Society;* and *Journal of General Microbiology.*

I should also like to thank the following for so kindly sparing me some of their valuable time for interviews: Professor Sir Ernst Chain, Dr. N.G. Heatley, Professor Charles Fletcher, Dr. Howard Hughes, Dr. A.J. Bard, Dr. L.M. Miall of Pfizer, Dr. J.H.C. Nayler of Beecham's, Dr. G.N. Rolinson and Mr. F. Batchelor of Beecham's, and Mr. H.W. Palmer of Glaxo.

In Search of
PENICILLIN

Chapter 1
PENICILLIN

THE STANDARD VERSION of the penicillin story is this: penicillin, the first of the antibiotic drugs. First observed by Sir Alexander Fleming in 1928 when he noticed that a stray mold had killed germs on one of his culture plates. Developed by Lord Florey and Professor Sir Ernst Chain at Oxford in 1940. Mass produced by the U.S. pharmaceutical industry, it saved the lives of thousands of Allied servicemen and came into world use after the end of World War II.

In Britain there is an addition to this story, for penicillin is widely held to be the supreme example of a national failing, the inability of the country's industrial technology to take advantage of, and reap the profit from, the discoveries of the scientists in its laboratories. It is widely believed that Britain lost, or gave up, the patents on penicillin to America and has since paid many millions of dollars to U.S. drug companies for the antibiotic. While no single item of this story is positively untrue, the whole adds up to a myth.

Fleming misinterpreted and misunderstood what he saw on his laboratory plate. He never found what was causing the effect he saw and never showed that his "penicillin" had any therapeutic or curative effect.

Florey and Chain did indeed develop penicillin into a drug in their Oxford laboratories, but this was not what they had set out to do at the start of their research program. Professor Howard Florey, an Australian physiologist appointed to the Professorship of Pathology in the ancient University was building up a new type of interdisciplinary team when he recruited the German-Jewish refugee biochemist, Ernst Chain. Together the two men proposed a program of purely scientific investigation into the phenomenon of bacterial antagonism, and, in the early stages of the work, came across Fleming's observation reported in the scientific literature ten years previously and virtually forgotten by 1938. The possibility that penicillin might have curative properties in man emerged still later in their research. Gradually it began to dominate their work and they recruited more and more people into the tasks of isolating, analyzing, manufacturing and testing the first antibiotic. The Oxford team slowly increased in size as more help became necessary, and Florey himself was always keen to credit the team rather than individuals. Gardner, Abraham and Heatley were among the earliest recruits to this team who figure largely in the story of penicillin.

Penicillin would almost certainly not be allowed to come onto the market if it was "discovered" today. Bodies such as the F.D.A. in America or the Medicines Commission in Britain would advise against it on account of the frequency of allergic side-effects. Penicillin might never have been developed at all if guinea pigs, which are badly affected by the drug, instead of mice had been the first experimental animals on which it was tested.

Mass production of penicillin was carried out in Britain and

Canada as well as the U.S., nor was it the American pharmaceutical industry only which showed how to obtain the most efficient production. There were no patents on penicillin because it was considered unethical for a scientist to patent a therapeutic discovery. Britain now sells penicillin-type drugs in the U.S. and obtains millions of dollars annually for the privilege of doing so.

The greatest distortion of the truth comes simply from presenting the story in a chronological order. This implies that progress toward the development of the first antibiotic drug, and hence the whole range of modern drugs, was logical and purposive. Scientists, and most of the rest of us, have been brought up to believe that there is a steady build-up of knowledge and experimentation from the first observation of biological activity, until the final product is marketed. This was certainly not the process in the case of penicillin which was marked throughout its story by the effects of luck, both bad and good, and sheer chance. And we still do not know, to this day, precisely how penicillin works.

Finally, the standard myth leaves out the most important thing about penicillin, which is the effect that its discovery, and development for therapeutic use, has had upon our modes of thought and our ways of looking at the world in which we find ourselves.

Go back to the very first word of the standard myth— penicillin. It is used in the singular, as it will be throughout this book. Yet this is incorrect, the word should be in the plural— penicillins. There are many different types of penicillin in nature and literally thousands more penicillins have been produced by scientists in their laboratories.

Penicillins are produced in nature by many different types of mold. Everyone knows what molds look like—they can be found on jam and bread, on boots and wood and carpets that have got wet. Scientifically the molds are living creatures of the same broad group as the fungi, and they are therefore related to the edible mushrooms that we eat. Their basic pattern of life is that they grow as a huge tangle of very fine threads. At intervals of time they produce fruiting bodies. Our edible mushrooms are examples of these. The fruiting bodies shed millions of spores, which are the reproductive seeds of the organism, into the atmosphere. These spores are too small to be seen with the naked eye, and they are extremely light, so they are carried by the wind along with the myriads of particles of plant pollen and they are to be found in all the air we breathe.

When a spore lands, by chance, on a hospitable medium it germinates and starts producing the fine threads which make up the main body of a new mold. To grow, it takes in nutrients from the medium in which it finds itself, like any other living organism, and similarly it produces by-products of this normal metabolic process. The penicillins are by-products of the life of various species of molds—the *Penicillium* molds, some of the molds of the *Aspergillus* family and the molds of the type called *Cephalosporium.*

The original penicillin was produced by a mold of the *Penicillium* family, which gets its name from the Latin word for brush, because the fruiting bodies of this type of mold, which can only be seen under the microscope, look like tiny paintbrushes. They exude their spores from the end of the bristles.

There are at least 650 species of molds classified as *Penicillium,* and there are many different strains within most of the species. There are, therefore, several thousand different penicillium molds, and what is even more complicating, most of the strains produce mutants easily and comparatively often.

It is now known that any particular penicillium mold can produce, by itself, several different types of penicillin as by-products of its normal life-process. The proportions of the different types of penicillin produced by any one mold will vary according to the medium on which it is growing. In other words, if you feed the creature on a particular diet it will produce more or less of a certain type of penicillin.

But among the many varieties of penicillium molds there are those which naturally produce higher proportions of one type of penicillin or another, and the scientist or chemical engineer who wishes to obtain one particular type of penicillin will have to search for the variety of mold which produces that particular type of penicillin in the highest proportion.

To understand this state of affairs more clearly it is necessary to grasp the chemical nature of penicillins. All penicillins consist of two parts, a nucleus and a side-chain. The chemists describe penicillins as "a nucleus containing a thiazolidine ring fused to a beta-lactam ring to which is attached a side-chain." The molecule of penicillin can be thought of as looking like this:

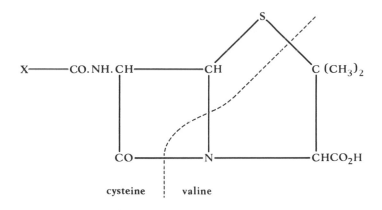

In this diagram S stands for an atom of sulphur, N for an atom of nitrogen, C for carbon, H for hydrogen and O for an atom of oxygen. It can be seen that some of the atoms occur by themselves whereas sometimes they are in groups as, for instance, at the bottom right-hand corner where we have $CHCO_2H$, which some chemists prefer to write as CH.COOH. These groups of atoms are all formations which are well known to the chemist since they are frequently found in nature and occur regularly as groups, as substructures of other compounds; they have an internal shape of their own but they regularly join up as part of other larger structures, such as the penicillin molecule.

The thiazolidine ring is the five-sided structure, like the

end view of a house in a child's drawing, on the right-hand side. The black lines indicate that there are chemical bonds, or attractive forces, between the atoms and groups of atoms. There are also repulsive forces between atoms as a general rule, and the combination of the various attractive and repulsive forces gives the molecule its shape. In real life the molecule of penicillin does not lie flat in one plane as shown on the paper, but has bends and wiggles which give it a shape in three dimensions.

The beta-lactam ring is the square on the left side of the drawing which shares one wall with the thiazolidine ring. These two rings together are the nucleus of all penicillins; and the two rings together, without anything else stuck on, are called 6-amino-penicillanic acid, or 6-APA.

The third feature of the structure is marked as X.CO. This is the side-chain and X can be a wide variety of substances, most of them perfectly well known in their own right. The traditional chemical diagram, as in the illustration, is rather deceptive because there is often more of the side-chain than there is of the nucleus. In the commonest medical form of penicillin (penicillin G or benzylpenicillin) the side-chain consists of fourteen more atoms of carbon and hydrogen, written by chemists as $C_6H_5CH_2$. This signifies a chain of six carbon atoms linked together in a line; five of them have hydrogen atoms linked to them and the sixth has the CH_2 substructure linked to it. The whole of this joins on to the top left-hand group of atoms in the beta-lactam ring of the penicillin nucleus.

The two-ring structure of penicillin was something unique in nature as far as the first investigators of penicillin were concerned; it was a structure they had never come across before. But it was not extraordinary, in the sense that it could be seen to be a joining up of two quite well-known constituents. For all that the penicillin nucleus looks like two rings in the diagram, it can equally well be regarded as two structures divided by the dashed line on the illustration.

The structure of atoms on the left-hand side of the dashed

line form a molecule of the substance cysteine, and the part to the right-hand side is then seen to be a molecule of valine. Valine and cysteine are both amino-acids, and the amino-acids are the building blocks of the enzymes and proteins which are essential parts of our bodies and, indeed, with a few additions, of virtually all bacterial and animal life. In principle, therefore, there is nothing very unusual about penicillin. It consists of two of the basic building blocks of living matter, joined up in a way which is not common and which is apparently only achieved in the course of normal life by certain species of molds.

The different behaviors of the different penicillins are governed entirely by the nature of the side-chains. It is because they have different side-chains that different penicillins are active in different strength against different bacteria and bacilli. For instance, right at the start of Florey's work it seemed clear that penicillin could not be given to patients by mouth because it was so unstable when acids were present.

But eventually scientists were able to produce penicillins which could be taken by mouth, simply by finding a side-chain which was active against germs but which also protected the nucleus against the attacks of acids. Many side-chains give penicillins which are completely useless as drugs and which do not attack bacteria at all.

The strange thing is that the side-chains, viewed as substances in their own right, do not usually possess any antibacterial activity. They only kill bacteria when they are attached to the penicillin nucleus. Yet the nucleus itself has very little activity against bacteria if it is stripped of its side-chain. Furthermore, the nucleus is rendered quite useless if any of the vital chemical links of its two rings are broken. There are a good many links in the penicillin molecule, as the diagram shows, and there are therefore a good many places in which the structure can be broken. A broken nucleus, even with its side-chain still attached, is powerless against bacteria. There are a very large number of breakdown products of penicillin: penicillamine and penillic acid, penillamine, penicilloic acid, penicillenic acid, penillonic acid, the penillo-aldehydes and so on. The differences between these breakdown products depend largely upon which link or bond in the penicillin nucleus has been broken.

The structure of penicillin, therefore, hardly explains its action. Indeed the situation seems highly illogical, for we know that penicillin kills germs, yet the penicillins consist of side-chains which are by themselves quite incapable of killing germs, and a nucleus which is barely capable of killing germs. Yet any damage to the nucleus renders the whole powerless to affect bacteria or bacilli. And the truth of the matter is that we do not know, even now, the full and final details of how penicillin works.

The first clue to the mode of operation of penicillin against bacteria came very early in the story, as far back as 1940. And it was overlooked for years. But Arthur D. Gardner (later Professor), a member of Florey's small group at Oxford, had shown that bacteria treated with very small doses of penicillin, so that they were not actually killed, developed into rather odd and gigantic shapes. Some of the bacteria, when viewed under the microscope seemed, indeed, to grow into enormous sizes when given very small amounts of penicillin.

It was not until 1946 that the first suggestion was made that penicillin might act by damaging the cell walls of the bacteria, a suggestion which would explain the strange shapes found by Gardner. But this was admitted to be pure speculation, and another ten years had to pass before it was widely accepted that penicillin works by acting specifically on the cell walls of bacteria.

The outside wall, the cell wall, of a bacterium consists of two parts. There is a flexible bag which holds in the chemicals such as enzymes and the genetic material that are needed by the creature. It can be thought of as a rubbery balloon which keeps liquids in or out. This rubber balloon is protected and held in shape by a more rigid outer structure which is, however, easily passed by chemicals and liquids. Two of the essential components of this outer structure are large molecules called muramic acid and teichoic acid. It's quite useful to think of them as two different types of steel girder each used over and over again to form an entire, regular structure.

Penicillin kills a bacterium by getting itself attached to this outer structure when it is being built, and somehow stopping the building up of the pieces of muramic acid. Large quantities of unused alanine, an amino-acid which is one of the building blocks of muramic acid, can be found inside a growing bacterium which is being attacked by penicillin. The ruination of the outer structure of the cell wall leaves the inner bag unprotected and unsupported. The osmotic pressure inside the bag then bursts it; the contents spill out, and the bacterium is dead. It is possible that the presence of penicillin also helps in some way to weaken or break the inner bag, but the main effect is the prevention of the construction of the outer wall.

It is likely, therefore, that penicillins achieve their effects partly because of their shape and partly because of the chemical activity of their constituents. There must be something about the shape of the penicillins (probably some feature of the shape of the nucleus) that enables them to fit physically into the structure of the bacterial cell wall; yet they must also be chemically more attractive to the other components of the wall than those materials like muramic acid which go into the building of the normal wall. Presumably also the penicillins in some way are more chemically attractive to the components of muramic acid than those components are to each other, since the components appear to be manufactured properly by the bacteria but are not joined up to make the normal acid.

This description of the action of penicillin accounts satisfactorily for the observed differences in the effectiveness of penicillin against different types of bacteria. Indeed, it is in many respects deduced from, or was discovered through, the differences in effectiveness.

Bacteria differ among themselves and they differ in the construction of their cell walls. One of these differences concerns the relative proportions of teichoic and muramic acids used in the construction of the cell walls. And, broadly speaking, penicillin is most effective in dealing with those bacteria which have the highest proportion of muramic acid in their cell walls.

From the early days of bacteriology in the nineteenth century it has been common to divide bacteria into two large groups, those which are Gram-positive and those which are Gram-negative. This distinction means no more than that Gram-positive bacteria will take up a chemical staining liquid which makes them more easily visible under the microscope. This useful chemical dye was discovered by the Danish scientist Hans Gram in 1884. But right from the start of the penicillin story it was discovered that penicillin was effective against Gram-positive bacteria, and at first it seemed that it simply did not work against Gram-negative germs. It has since been shown that penicillin has some effect against almost every known type of bacterium, though sometimes such large doses are required to stop the progress of certain Gram-negative bacteria that its use in clinical treatment would be quite impracticable. Gram-positive organisms cause most local septic infections, septicemia, puerperal fever, osteomyelitis, anthrax, tuberculosis, diphtheria, tetanus and pneumonia. Gram-negative organisms include the germs of plague, cholera, typhoid, and food poisoning.

The crucial work in explaining the activity of penicillin was performed as recently as 1956 when it was shown that Gram-positive bacteria differ from Gram-negative bacteria largely in the proportions of the building materials in their cell walls. It was also shown that all Gram-positive bacteria used muramic acid as part of their cell wall structure. Nevertheless, when the thirtieth anniversary of the first cures achieved by penicillin was celebrated in 1971 by an international scientific symposium at the Royal Society in London, Dr. J.L. Strominger of Harvard was one of the chief speakers and his paper was entitled "How penicillin kills bacteria: progress and problems." This made it quite clear that the final answers to the question have not yet been achieved.

There are, however, two most important corollaries to be

drawn out of this description of the structure and mode of action of the penicillins. The first is that penicillin does not, in strict terms, kill germs, though under the special conditions of scientific experiments in laboratory glassware it can be persuaded to do so. Normally penicillin does not attack bacteria that are fully grown or in a resting state. Instead it stops the growth of new bacteria by preventing them from constructing themselves properly. It attacks bacteria only when they are multiplying or reproducing themselves. In simple single-cell creatures like bacteria, reproduction occurs by division, where one bacterium grows and splits into two identical creatures. The common misunderstanding—that penicillin kills germs—stretches right back to the misinterpretation of Fleming's original discovery.

The second important corollary is that multicellular organizations, and notably animals and man, do not have the double structure in their cell walls. Our cells have as their containment a single rubber bag outer skin, and do not need the rigid steel-lattice extra structure that the single-celled bacteria have developed through the course of evolution. We do not use teichoic and muramic acids for constructing ourselves, nor do the animals.

This is the reason penicillins are not toxic to humans or animals in general. Penicillins do not stop us building anything we need, nor do they destroy human or animal cells. Now this was the aspect of penicillin that caused most surprise intellectually when it was first discovered—the fact that here was a substance which attacked bacterial cells and left human and animal cells unharmed. This was something which most scientists believed did not exist, something which attacked bacterial cells specifically. Before penicillin it had seemed that anything powerful enough to kill bacterial cells would at the same time attack the cells of the animal or man which was host to the bacteria. It was here that penicillin caused intellectual and social revolution and opened the way to our present society in which we positively expect the medical scientist to produce a cure for almost every disease by finding some chemical, drug, or mode of treatment, which will deal specifically with the cause of the disease condition.

Yet in the very act of presenting this review of penicillin as we know it now, the result of forty-five years of scientific work, I have distorted the story of penicillin. By the very process of looking backward through time, one puts the crucial discoveries that have led to our present view of the subject into a chronological perspective; a logic has been forced onto the history which did not exist at the time the discoveries were made. By writing "In 19—Jones found this and two years later Smith proved that," a logical connection is implied as linking the two events at that time. This is how scientists like to view the progress of their subjects. Certainly in the case of penicillin it was not like this.

The first patients to be cured by penicillin, in Oxford in 1941, were given what Florey and Chain believed at that time to be pure penicillin. We know now that only about two percent of the substance was penicillin and ninety-eight percent was impurities. And at the time that those patients were treated no one had any idea just what penicillin was. Indeed the final demonstration of the nature and structure of penicillin did not come until 1945, by which time hundreds of thousands of Allied and Axis servicemen had been treated with penicillin, and the drug was beginning to be widely used in civilian hospitals. There had even been attempts to manufacture it in secret by the Dutch underground and the French Maquis.

Of course the chemists in Professor Florey's small research group at Oxford had started trying to isolate, purify, and analyze penicillin right from the start. Chain was helped by the organic chemists, Sir Robert Robinson and Professor Wilson Baker, of the Oxford University Dyson Perrins Organic Chemistry Laboratory which was only a few hundred yards up the road from his own laboratory. Since they could not find a way of obtaining absolutely pure penicillin they started by working on the substances which resulted when penicillin was broken down chemically, something which happened all too easily for comfort in those early days. The first they found was the product named penicillamine (which has very recently proved to be a major boon to those suffering from serious arthritis). Unfortunately, in their chemical analysis of penicillamine they made a mistake and overlooked the presence of a sulphur atom in the penicillamine molecule. And when they found another breakdown product of penicillin, which is now called penillic acid, they made a similar error and again failed to spot a sulphur atom in its structure.

By the time these errors had been discovered and corrected American research laboratories had joined in the work. But at this moment scientific communication across the Atlantic broke down. In Britain the Official Secrets Act was applied to work on penicillin, and scientific publication was halted. In the U.S.A. much of the early work on penicillin was funded by the wartime Office of Scientific Research and Development, and under this contract workers in both commercial and academic laboratories were blocked from publishing their results. There was also commercial secrecy imposed on some of the industrial research in the U.S.

The problem was solved by the governments of the U.S.A. and the U.K. which agreed that, although all information on penicillin would remain an official secret and although secrecy on patents would be preserved, all information obtained on either side of the Atlantic under government auspices would be pooled and circulated on a need-to-know basis. This agreement worked surprisingly well considering the extraordinary way in which officialdom dealt with it. It was "An Agreement on the principles applying to the Exchange of Information relating to the Synthesis of Penicillin," which, in Britain, is Command Paper Number 6757, published by H.M.S.O. in 1946. It was not, in fact, finally ratified until 1946, some three months after it had expired, because the terms of the agreement state that it shall run from December 1, 1943 to October 31, 1945. However, it worked and information flowed.

The Oxford workers found the sulphur atoms they had missed and in late 1943 there was transatlantic agreement on the formula of penicillamine. But there continued to be a marked difference between British and American figures for the structure of penillic acid. Oxford continued to get the formula $C_{14}H_{20}O_4N_2S$, while the Americans found $C_{16}H_{18}O_4N_2S$. This difference of results was only solved when it became clear that different penicillins were being made in different proportions on the two sides of the Atlantic. Before the end of the war at least four different penicillins were being produced and had been identified. The British called them penicillins I, II, III and IV, with some appearance of logicality; the Americans named them penicillins G, F, K and X with less system, but the American naming has prevailed. There was obviously considerable scientific confusion caused by the appearances of different penicillins, and much work in separating them out and establishing the correspondences between British and American varieties. The important one of these first four penicillins was penicillin G, technically benzylpenicillin, which is used in the medical profession to this day in very large quantities, and which was the original penicillin which went on the market as the first of the antibiotic drugs.

The first people to suggest what turned out to be the correct structure of penicillin, "a nucleus containing a thiazolidine ring fused to a beta-lactam ring to which is attached a side-chain," were Chain and Abraham in Oxford. This was in 1943. But they were not able to prove their claim at that time. Two more years had to pass before the Americans produced the first crystals of really pure penicillin from which final and definitive proof of the nature of the molecule could be obtained. It must be remembered that the ability to purify and analyze complex molecules produced by living matter was, at that time, at the very frontiers of science; indeed one of the major efforts of all chemists and biochemists right up to the present is to identify, analyze and determine the precise mode of action of the very large molecules which make up living creatures. The final analysis of the chemical structure of penicillin was completed at Oxford in 1946 by the x-ray analysis of pure penicillin crystals produced by the American laboratories. By this time the war was over and penicillin was in large-scale production for world use.

When penicillin was introduced into general medical use at the end of the war the British Pharmaceutical Council published a technical book for the instruction of its members and for doctors and chemists. The problems facing those who had attempted to unravel the mysteries of penicillin were well summed up:

> Attempts to determine the structure of an organic compound are generally made only after it has been prepared in the pure state, but the chemical constitution of the penicillins was investigated long before the crystalline substances had been obtained. In fact some of the early results which laid down the foundations of our present knowledge were obtained with material that contained more impurities than it did penicillin, which was itself a mixture of several closely related substances.

It was only the development of methods for mass production of penicillin as a drug that made enough pure penicillin available for the laboratory chemists to complete their analysis of the structure. The same availability of large quantities of penicillin for research work brought a definite confusion to the parallel scientific problem of finding out how penicillin worked.

Looking back, the trail seems fairly clear up to about 1946. Fleming had first been interested in the substance because it caused lysis of the bacteria on his culture plate—that is, the bacteria appeared to have been killed by being broken open. We have seen that Gardner, in Oxford, had noted the odd and gigantic shapes achieved by bacteria treated with very small amounts of penicillin and that it had been suggested that penicillin achieved its effects by acting against the walls of the bacterial cells. All this work had been done on Gram-positive bacteria which were the types of bacteria attacked by penicillin, while it was known from Fleming's original work that penicillin did not attack Gram-negative organisms.

But with the availability of large quantities of penicillin for research purposes, tests were now carried out on almost every known organism of disease, using enormously large or alternatively very small doses of the drug. It was shown that penicillin could, under certain circumstances, attack Gram-negative bacteria; likewise it appeared that at very small doses its effect upon Gram-positive organisms varied from one to another. Penicillin resistance also appeared, and organisms like staphylococci which differed in no outward way from those which had been slaughtered by penicillin were now found to be able to stand up to large doses of the antibiotic. We know now that this is because mutants of these organisms are capable of producing penicillinase, a natural substance which splits up the nucleus of penicillin, but when the phenomenon of penicillin resistance first appeared it was extremely difficult to understand.

In effect such understanding as we possess of the mode of action of penicillin had to await the development of techniques for studying the cell walls of bacteria in their chemical make-up and in their three-dimensional structure. It was to take a further ten years of work over very broad areas of scientific advance before it could be shown that the cell walls of different bacteria contained differing proportions of building blocks and give the clue about the importance of muramic acid.

And this line of approach is still not concluded. There is still no final agreement about how penicillin works. There is, however, an interesting shift of emphasis. It is common now to find scientists treating penicillin, about which we know a great deal, as a valuable tool to probe into the much wider and more important subject of the construction and mode of behavior of bacteria.

Chapter 2
BACKGROUND

THE STORY OF PENICILLIN begins with Louis Pasteur. But then, so much of modern medicine begins with Pasteur—antiseptics and antiseptic surgery, bacteriology, immunology, epidemiology, public health, immunization programs as well as antibiotics.

This was merely 110 years ago. Modern medicine was founded only at the time of the American Civil War.

Faced with any disease, we automatically ask: How did this come about? Is there a causative organism? What germ or virus has caused it? Indeed it is those diseases, like cancer and rheumatism that do not have obvious causal organisms, which most baffle us. And beyond questions of our own health and comfort we are aware of the world of micro-organisms. We know that there are invisible creatures in air and water, in the soil and the plants and the animals, that are living and breeding, competing with us, even when they don't actually harm us.

It is almost impossible to project the human imagination back to a time when these things were unknown, even unthought of.

It was Pasteur who was responsible for proving the germ theory of infectious and transmissible diseases. It was he who showed that infectious diseases were caused by the invasion and multiplication within our bodies of invisible but living creatures. This is the medical way of looking at his work. More important was the revolution in thought that Pasteur produced; the revolution that made us aware of the existence of all the myriads of creatures of the micro-world alongside our own macro-world; the revolution that provided a rationale for most diseases and epidemics and therefore allowed the rational development of treatments against the diseases or the acquisition of protection against microbial invasion.

Pasteur was essentially a chemist and a veterinarian. His own work was almost entirely limited to animals because he did not have medical qualifications. It was in 1864 that he proved that the process of fermentation, known to man for thousands of years, was in essence the action of living creatures, the yeasts. He had been called in, as a chemist, to troubleshoot some production problems in a friend's vinegar factory.

He showed that the globules in the fermentation vats were living creatures; that the fermentation occurred as a result of their life processes. He then demonstrated that each type of fermentation was the result of the action of particular and different yeasts. From this he went on to show that yeasts could also produce the type of acid found in sour milk, and hence he concluded that all spoiling and putrefaction was caused by living organisms which were all about us in the air and dust. This led to a series of experiments in which he showed that meat and broths would not be rotted and spoiled as long as air was excluded from them. This, in turn, led him to invent various ways, including heating, by which the micro-organisms could be killed. By demonstrating how things could be preserved he also showed that the air was full of living organisms which attacked meats, sugars and so on.

On the one hand this led to the whole system of pasteurization and the preservation of food by heating and thence to the modern canning and packaging industries. On the other hand, his observations were taken up by Lister, the great Scottish surgeon, who argued that if the air was full of living, spoiling, putrefying organisms, the killing of these organisms would prevent the infection of surgical wounds which made all operations and amputations so dangerous. Lister's antiseptic surgery brought about a most dramatic decrease in the rate of death from operating wounds, and from 1865 onward revolutionized medical, and especially surgical, practice. The application of antiseptic techniques under the influence of Pasteur's disciples in the maternity hospitals vastly reduced the casualties from puerperal or childbed fever.

The philosophical revolution wrought here by Pasteur was probably even more important, for he finally demolished the theories of spontaneous generation held by many distinguished scientists and bitterly conservative medical men. He proved that life only sprang from life and was not the result of the combination of non-living matter in suitable circumstances and environments. This may seem obvious to us, but Pasteur demolished long-held beliefs, based often on observations by reputable scientists, or natural philosophers as they considered themselves, that bees and beetles could be produced by cow dung. This is not to say that Pasteur produced all the experimental results or scientific observations himself. He was personally responsible for many of the most exciting scientific discoveries of his time, but there were many others who observed microbes and successfully investigated diseases or ferments, most notably Robert Koch in Germany who discovered the bacillus (the germ) of anthrax, the dreaded disease of cattle and sheep which sometimes affects man. But Pasteur had an exceptional authority and weight in public debate, not only because of his brilliant personal successes, but even more because of his ability to demonstrate by experiment, to prove publicly and convince the doubters.

It cannot be without significance that Pasteur was a great

influence on the three men who did most to bring penicillin to the world. Both Fleming and Florey often quoted him, and Chain openly regards him as the greatest of all scientists and decorates his study with aphorisms pronounced by Pasteur.

After his successes in fermenting and brewing research, Pasteur was called to help with a problem of disease among silkworms and went on to work on the disease of chicken cholera. He successfully identified and isolated the bacteria causing the disease, proving his point by growing the bacteria in cultures of chicken-gristle broth and infecting fresh chickens with the disease by inoculating them with the bacteria from the broth.

The greatest and happiest accident came about because Pasteur had gone away on a short holiday and had left his plates of chicken-cholera bacteria unattended. On his return the work started again and chickens were injected with bacteria from these stale plates. To his annoyance these chickens failed to develop the disease. Fresh cultures of bacteria were therefore grown and injected into the chickens. Those chickens which had been injected with the stale cultures still did not develop cholera when injected with fresh bacteria, whereas chickens which had not received injections with the stale culture died rapidly from the disease. Pasteur, author of the phrase "Chance only favors the prepared mind," saw what it meant. By chance he had attenuated the bacteria, deprived them of their virulence. The stale bacteria had given the chickens something like a very mild version of the cholera and left them immune to attacks by the normal virulent bacteria.

His discovery correlated with something well known to medical men, indeed to most men, for many thousands of years: once a person recovered from an infectious disease—measles, smallpox or the plague—he very rarely contracted the same disease again. Furthermore, Pasteur's findings gave a scientific rationale to one of the very few real medical advances ever achieved before his time: Jenner's vaccination.

From ancient times the Chinese and Arabs had developed the practice of taking scrapings from mild cases of smallpox and infecting the healthy with these scrapings in the hope that they, too, would have only a mild case of the disease, and would remain little marked and immune for the rest of their lives. Voltaire claimed that this practice reached its highest perfection among the mountain-dwelling Circassians, for their only export commodity was their beautiful daughters who could not be sold to the harems of the rich if they were marked by the pocks of the disease. The practice was introduced to Western Europe largely by Lady Mary Wortley Montagu, wife of an eighteenth-century British ambassador to Constantinople. It was adopted by the Hanoverian kings of England after it had been tried out on some convicts and orphan children, and some historians suggest that the reduction of deaths from smallpox was one of the causes of the British population growth which provided the necessary substrate for the start of the Industrial Revolution.

Edward Jenner, a Gloucestershire doctor, took the process of protection against smallpox an important stage further by using material collected from the sores of milkmaids suffering from cowpox, a comparatively mild disease, to inoculate as a preventive against smallpox. He proved his point on a young boy, inoculating him with cowpox germs and then infecting the child with virulent smallpox material to demonstrate that the inoculation had provided real protection   proof indeed, but availing himself of a more robust ethic than we would allow nowadays. Jenner named his procedure vaccination from the Latin word for cow, *vacca*. His later life was filled with controversy but he became the first human being ever to show how to defeat an infectious disease on a rational basis. William Pitt used his great powers of oratory to sway the House of Commons to reward Jenner for work which is still the basis of our present-day protection against smallpox. The Royal College of Physicians would never grant Jenner membership because he could not pass an examination in Latin. But Pasteur kept to the word vaccination, to describe his much more sophisticated procedures of preventive inoculation, in honor of Jenner.

It was shown that it was exposure to the oxygen of the air that had attenuated the virulence of the chicken-cholera bacteria. So the process could easily be repeated on a large scale and there was no problem in making large quantities of the vaccine and virtually wiping out the disease. The conquest of anthrax was Pasteur's next great triumph. The bacillus had been discovered and identified by Robert Koch, but it was Pasteur who confirmed and publicly demonstrated the merit of Koch's work by cultivating the bacillus in the laboratory and showing that it caused the disease when injected into healthy animals. He eventually discovered how to attenuate the germ, by heat, and thus was able to prepare a vaccine. The effectiveness of the vaccine was demonstrated by a great public experiment at Pouilly-le-Fort just outside Paris. No fewer than 25 sheep, 6 oxen and an odd goat were vaccinated in public. A few days later they were equally publicly inoculated with preparations of anthrax bacteria along with 25 sheep, 4 cows and another goat that had not been given protective vaccination. After a rather worrying few days, during which one or two of the protected animals showed some disturbing symptoms, yet another public gathering of doctors, vets, variegated scientists, farmers, administrators and even peasants, saw that all the unprotected animals were dead of anthrax or in the last throes of the disease, while all those vaccinated protectively were thoroughly healthy. This occurred in June 1881.

Because Pasteur had no medical qualification he had been forced to confine himself to research on animal diseases. Presumably it was his election to the Académie de Médecine as well as the Académie Française that allowed him to turn to a disease which is as fatal for humans as for animals.

His final conquest was of hydrophobia, also called rabies, which is transmitted to humans usually by the bite of a mad dog. Pasteur never identified the causative organism. We know now that it is a virus too small to be seen under anything but the electron microscope. But he proved that there must be a transmissible organism which eventually lodges in the brain of the infected creature, and he prepared a vaccine by drying the spinal cords of infected rabbits. Because rabies is so slow to develop after the infection by bite, Pasteur hoped to protect those bitten by a rabid animal by giving them injections after they had been infected yet before the disease had developed. He showed that this protection was possible when a dog was bitten by a rabid dog, and the story of his eventual success in proving the application to humans by treating nine-year-old Joseph Meister, who was brought to him by distraught parents all the way from Alsace, is quite well known. What is less known is that this same Joseph Meister eventually became porter and gatekeeper at the Institut Pasteur in Paris and committed suicide when the German invaders wished to enter the crypt containing Pasteur's remains in 1940.

It was Pasteur's final triumph: the ability to protect nearly everyone who had been bitten by a rabid animal as long as the patient got to him in time. People flocked to Paris and Pasteur from all over the world. Despite the length of the trip, American children were brought across the Atlantic by boat; a group of Russian peasants, ravaged by a mad wolf that had terrorized their village, arrived only able to utter the word Pasteur. Enough of the Russians went back eventually to persuade the Czar to be one of the largest subscribers to the setting up of the Institut Pasteur, which was built for research and to conduct the service of inoculation against rabies.

Before Pasteur died in 1895, the microbes causing plague and diphtheria had been identified and research was in progress to find the organisms causing yellow fever, tuberculosis and cholera. The approach to all these diseases was the same. First the causative organism must be identified, and Pasteur had shown how this could be demonstrated definitively out of the many possible candidates for incrimination among the multitude of micro-organisms found in the bodies of dead sufferers. The organism had to be cultivated in some medium outside the body and then it had to produce the disease when re-injected into healthy animals. In a sense he had been driven into this clarity of expression by his many opponents who time and again would claim that it was some other, unidentified factor in the blood or the air or the soil that really caused the disease.

This demonstrative process was similar to the process for obtaining attenuated strains of the microbes suitable for protective inoculation. For the microbes, bacteria or bacilli grown in laboratory cultures could be experimented upon, using heat or light or exposure to oxygen in the search for attenuation mechanisms.

The results of this method were the production of what we now call live attenuated vaccines. In these vaccines a non-virulent or attenuated strain of the causative organism, whether it is bacterium or virus, is injected into healthy people, to stimulate their defenses and render them immune to any later attack by virulent organisms of that kind. The alternative to this type of vaccine is the killed vaccine in which virulent germs of the normal disease-causing organism are killed and then injected into those who desire protection. Our present knowledge shows that killed vaccines give much shorter times of immunity, perhaps only three months' protection, whereas the live attenuated vaccines usually give lifelong immunity, but carry some margin of danger in that the attenuated strain of organism can either be contaminated with virulent organisms during manufacture or can itself mutate back into a virulent type.

These vaccines, however, are only part of the immunological armory that Pasteur and his disciples gave to medicine. They confer active immunity on the recipient, which means that they activate the body's natural defenses against a potential invader. But there is also passive immunity by which the natural defense mechanisms (the nature of which were unknown to Pasteur) manufactured by one body can be transferred, by injection, to a second body which is actually under attack. In the 1880s, as developed by Pasteur's collaborator, Dr. Emile Roux, this meant that horses were injected with diphtheria bacilli, allowed to manufacture the natural defense against the microbe, and then this natural defense could be extracted from the horse blood-serum and injected into humans suffering from an attack of diphtheria. In the case of diphtheria, Roux understood that the damage to the human body was actually caused by a toxic substance produced by the germ as it grew. And he understood that the unknown substance obtained from the horse was an antitoxin which neutralized the product of the diphtheria germ. Nevertheless it seemed that it would also be possible to produce from the bodies of animals both antitoxins against the products of invading bacteria and substances that would act against the bacteria themselves. For some diseases we still use vaccines manufactured in the bodies of living animals, smallpox being the most obvious example, but we also know about the dangers involved. In Pasteur's later years it seemed that serotherapy must have a future of promise as great as that facing immunization.

Pasteur's successful demonstration of the germ theory of infectious disease stimulated the fields of public health and hygiene, in addition to antiseptic surgery. The belief that a good water supply is the basis of public health sprang from his demonstrations of germs in water, and the second half of the nineteenth century was studded with public controversies, law suits and scientific discoveries concerning water supplies.

Pasteur, in fact, set the course that medicine would take for the seventy years from his first great discoveries up to 1940. This course depended upon immunology as the chief weapon in defeating infectious diseases and used serotherapy as virtually the only known way of dealing with bacteria which had successfully invaded the body.

This line of progress continues to the present day. The great early triumphs of immunology were the discoveries of vaccines against yellow fever, cholera, typhus and so on. This phase of development reached its climax in the development and application of vaccination against diphtheria in the 1930s. Penicillin and the antibiotics opened up a different approach to curing disease, but in our own post-war era, immunology has had to continue in the old way to deal with those diseases, mostly diseases caused by viruses, which are not affected by antibiotics. The production of vaccine against poliomyelitis is one of the great successes of our time, but it is only within the last ten years that we have produced vaccines against measles and, perhaps more important, vaccines against rubella (i.e., German measles) which we use now not so much to protect ourselves from the disease but to protect the yet unconceived children who could so easily be damaged if their mothers should suffer from this disease during pregnancy.

Yet throughout the early years of immunology, when plague, anthrax, yellow fever and the great scourges of mankind were being controlled, the medical scientists who developed the new vaccines had no idea of how they worked. Pasteur himself at first favored the theory that the protective vaccine used up or absorbed some factor in the body which was necessary for the later growth of a virulent invader. Later in his life he switched to a rather vague belief that the protective vaccine introduced some factor which combated any later invasion.

Our present knowledge of the immune defense systems of the body pictures the whole scene as "the science of self." We see our bodies as having a mechanism, carried in the white cells of the bloodstream called lymphocytes, which enables each individual body to recognize those cells which are its own and tolerate them, and likewise to recognize any cell which is not its own and attack it. Every cell carries on its surface chemical substances called antigens which are in some way an expression of the genetic material which is the core of the cell. It is these antigens which are recognized by lymphocytes. When lymphocytes recognize an antigen as being not-self they do two things; they multiply themselves and they produce substances called antibodies, chemicals which attack the not-self cell by adhering to the antigen.

More than this, however, the vital part of modern immunological theory holds that one lymphocyte will recognize and produce antibody against one, and only one, type of antigen. Lymphocyte and antibody are specific to one antigen only. Yet a normal healthy body contains lymphocytes which can recognize every single antigen produced by any other creature in nature. Indeed when chemists produce an entirely new antigen, never found in nature, the body has a lymphocyte and antibody ready to deal with the synthetic antigen.

According to this theory, then, a protective inoculation with attenuated anthrax germs attracts those lymphocytes which are equipped with the power to bring about the production of anti-anthrax antibody, since the antigen on the outside of an attenuated anthrax germ is no different from that of a virulent germ. The same reaction is secured by the injection of dead, but undamaged, cholera germs. The reaction against the protective vaccine is vastly to increase the amount of antibody against that strain of bacteria and, more importantly, to multiply those lymphocytes which recognize and react against anthrax or cholera germs. And it is the persistence of large numbers of these particular lymphocytes in the bloodstream that confers immunity when the virulent germ attacks.

None of this was known in Pasteur's day and, indeed, most of it has been discovered only in the last twenty years. Nevertheless, despite their ignorance about the basic principles of the process, the medical scientists of the last years of the nineteenth century proceeded very successfully in the identification of the micro-organisms which caused the great disease scourges of mankind. And they produced vaccine after vaccine which controlled these diseases by protecting and immunizing men against infection. Not surprisingly, in view of success after success, the whole trend of medical thinking came to place more and more emphasis on immunological and sero-therapeutic techniques. This trend of thought was strengthened in France and many other countries by the predominant feeling that "natural" cures and methods, employing the stratagems that nature employed, must be best.

The historic link between the burgeoning world of Pasteur's legacy to medicine and the start of the penicillin story is the development of a vaccine against typhoid fever. This success of immunological medicine was achieved in 1898 by Sir Almroth Wright, who had been professor of pathology at the British Army School of Medicine at Netley Hospital near Southampton since 1892. His vaccine was a killed vaccine which promised to be extremely important in the military field because typhoid, which was often fatal in those days, was a particular scourge of armies under active service conditions.

But producing the vaccine and demonstrating favorable results in India was not enough to convince the military authorities. At the start of the Boer War, Wright wanted to have all soldiers compulsorily vaccinated before they left for foreign service. The medical establishment would have none of it. Wright was only allowed to vaccinate volunteers and he got only 16,000 volunteers out of 320,000 soldiers. And furthermore the obstruction of the dugouts made it impossible to follow up the results of even the 16,000 voluntary injections. There is a story of a medical sergeant-orderly who, for every victim of typhoid brought in, filled in a form to state that the victim *had* been vaccinated on the grounds that "the fact that they've got it proves as they've been vaccinated." As to the reality of Wright's achievement it need only be said that his vaccine is, in all essentials, that which we use today.

So Wright resigned from the Army Medical Service, but not before his ferocious arguments in favor of his cause had created public controversy and private rancor. Nor did he let the cause drop even after his resignation. Ten years or so later his personal friendship with Lord Haldane, then Secretary of State for War, earned him a knighthood. The news of this honor came in a letter from Haldane which is alleged to have run on these lines. "Dear Wright, we must have your Typhoid Prophylactic for the Army but I have failed to convince the head man of the Army Medical Service of this. I have, therefore, got to build you up as a Public Figure, and the first step is to make you a knight. You won't like it, but it has to be. . . . Haldane."

To anyone who knows large organizations, and the British Army in particular, it will be obvious what fury and what enmity it would have caused to have a junior figure, and a scientist at that, circumventing the official channels and appealing over the heads of his superiors through his personal acquaintance with a cabinet minister, a mere politician. After his noisy departure from the army, Wright was appointed professor of pathology at St. Mary's Hospital, Paddington, in London. He stayed there until 1945, though he officially resigned as professor of pathology in 1908 to become the founder and director of the Inoculation Department of the hospital.

Wright's early work at St. Mary's Hospital greatly increased his scientific reputation, whatever his quarrels with the military authorities may have done to his professional chances. There were at that time two rival theories trying to account for the observed success of immunological medicine. One theory held that there were factors in the blood, produced by the action of protective vaccination, which resisted later invasion by virulent germs. These factors were, of course, real; they were the antibodies we have since discovered and identified. But around the turn of the century scientific techniques were not discriminating enough to isolate these substances and only their effects could be observed. However, it was possible to observe the activities of the white blood cells called phagocytes. These cells could be seen under the microscope engulfing bacteria and carrying away the invading germs. It was natural, therefore, to guess that protective vaccination fortified, or armed, or strengthened the phagocytes in some way and helped them perform the task of dealing with invasive organisms more efficiently. We know that the phagocytes are the cleaners and sweepers of our systems, carrying off any undesirable particles that get into our bloodstreams as well as clearing up natural debris from dead and broken cells. They can, indeed, engulf and carry off invading germs and bacteria but only after these organisms have been attacked by antibody. Wright's early work led directly to our modern views. He reconciled the two rival theories of immunological mechanism; he showed that there were factors circulating in the blood which increased the amount of phagocytosis, that is, the rapidity and avidity with which the white-cell phagocytes digest and carry away invading microbes.

This cooperation between what we now call antibodies in the blood stream and the phagocytes has become a well-established part of our modern understanding of the immune process and up to this point Wright had done good work. But from here he went rushing off in his enthusiastic, dogmatic and unchecked way on to various false tracks. The property acquired by the blood to reinforce the destructive action of the phagocytes he called opsonic and the substance itself he named opsonin. Both words are derived from the Greek *opsono* which means "I prepare food for . . ." This in itself was typical of Wright, he was a great advocate of the correct use of Greek and Latin roots for newly-coined medical words.

George Bernard Shaw, the playwright, became a personal friend of Sir Almroth Wright and often visited the research laboratories at St. Mary's Hospital. Wright's theories have, as a result, been immortalized in English literature, for Shaw's play *The Doctor's Dilemma* was in fact a description of the thinking and action that went on around Wright, and the character Sir Colenso Ridgeon is a very thinly disguised portrait of Wright himself. In the first act of the play Sir Colenso Ridgeon outlines his theories to the skeptical medical man of the older schools, Sir Patrick, and George Bernard Shaw writes this superb summary of Wright's theory:

> RIDGEON: Opsonin is what you butter the disease germs with to make your white corpuscles eat them. . . . what it comes to in practice is this. The phagocytes won't eat the microbes unless the microbes are nicely buttered for them. Well the patient manufactures the butter for himself all right; but my discovery is that the manufacture of that butter, which I call opsonin, goes on in the system by ups and downs—Nature being always rhythmical you know—and what the inoculation does is to stimulate the ups or downs as the case may be. . . . Inoculate when the patient is in the negative phase and you kill; inoculate when the patient is in the positive phase and you cure.

And that was exactly what Wright practiced at the Inoculation Department of St. Mary's Hospital. An allegedly quantitative measurement of the opsonic state of the patient's blood, the so-called opsonic index, was worked out and new and advanced techniques for finding and calculating the index were developed. On the basis of this index, treatments by the method of auto-vaccination were carried out—this involved finding what germ caused the boil or infection or sepsis, culturing it in the laboratory, preparing an antitoxin or killed vaccine from the germ and re-injecting this auto-vaccine into the patient.

Sir Almroth Wright dominated his department and the team of brilliant young men he gathered about him. A shambling, excitable, dogmatic, domineering, voluble creature: "one of the most remarkable men who ever entered medicine," according to Professor Ronald Hare who worked under him for several years. His father was an Irish Presbyterian, his mother the daughter of a Swedish professor of organic chemistry. He was a much more cosmopolitan figure than the average British medical man of his time: he had traveled widely in Europe and received much of his education on the Continent. His concept of a professor was the nineteenth-century German one of a complete lord of his department. He claimed that his department was "a republic," but the best that could be said of it was that it was "an enlightened despotism." His greatest love was poetry and he claimed that he could recite from memory some 250,000 lines from the Bible, Dante, Goethe, and the great English poets (including Kipling in the list). He loved literary academic conversation, the more high-flown the better.

But he was undoubtedly attractive. He had a passion for science and languages as well as for poetry. He learned Russian at sixty-two and in the last days of his life began the study of Eskimo. He had firm friends among the great scientists of Europe, notably Paul Ehrlich. He had influential friends among politicians, notably Balfour and Haldane. Above all he had friends in the brightest literary and artistic circles. Shaw was by no means the only regular visitor from the world of theater and gallery to the Inoculation Department.

And above all, Wright inspired devotion and enthusiasm among the brilliant young scientists he gathered around him at St. Mary's. Some of his pupils from Netley came with him when he left the army and moved to Paddington, and all of them made notable contributions to bacteriology. Sir William Leishman is probably the most famous. The young men he recruited when he reached St. Mary's are probably even more distinguished. At least four became Fellows of the Royal Society and another became a Fellow of the Royal Society of Canada, while many others became professors and directors of various institutes.

In his prime Wright worked tirelessly and he inspired the others to do so as well. But there is no doubt that he was extremely tiresome to work with and, to quote Professor Hare:

> He became a medical nuisance of the first order. He never missed an opportunity of pillorying Harley Street for its old-fashioned methods of medical practice, getting himself dubbed the "Prophet from Praed Street" by one of the medical journals for his pains. And towards the end of the First World War he succeeded in making himself thoroughly detested by most of the medical profession for publishing what can only be described as a masterpiece of sustained invective attacking the then President of the Royal College of Surgeons. It is perhaps not surprising that with such a person in charge, his laboratory was ruled with a rod of iron. Every member of the team had to support him and his somewhat revolutionary ideas wholeheartedly. The few who could not do so got out, but among those who accepted these conditions were some of the best brains in the profession.

Perhaps the most significant demonstration of Sir Almroth's dominance can be found in the fact that he wrote the entry on immunity in the 1922 edition of the *Encyclopaedia Britannica* and that he used this as an opportunity for expounding his opsonic theory in full. Yet before 1930 workers in his own department (notably Colebrook and Hare) had disproved the basis of these opsonic theories and shown that whatever the opsonic index measured it was certainly not what it was supposed to measure.

A department so full of talk, so full of theories, so full of brilliant scientists and famous visitors was, naturally, a leader of opinion, the center of a school of thought. In the case of the Inoculation Department at St. Mary's Hospital this, naturally again, was the immunological school of thought. And under Wright this developed a rather unscientific exclusiveness, a tendency to reject any other mode of thought but its own. We can turn best to George Bernard Shaw, that master of the English language, to see how his thinking expressed itself. In *The Doctor's Dilemma* Shaw expresses the philosophy of Wright through the mouth of Sir Ralph Bloomfield Bonington, the pompous, yet successful medico:

> Drugs can only repress symptoms; they cannot eradicate disease. The true remedy for all diseases is Nature's remedy. Nature and Science are at one, Sir Patrick, believe me; though you were taught differently. Nature has provided in the white corpuscles as you call them—in the phagocytes as we call them—a natural means of devouring and destroying all disease germs. There is at bottom only one genuinely scientific treatment of all diseases and that is to stimulate the phagocytes. Stimulate the phagocytes. Drugs are a delusion. Find the germ of the disease; prepare from it a suitable anti-toxin; inject it three times a day quarter of an hour before meals; and what is the result? The phagocytes are stimulated; they devour the disease; and the patient recovers—unless, of course, he's too far gone. That, I take it, is the essence of Ridgeon's discovery.

Sir Almroth Wright summed up his doctrine more succinctly in real life: "Mobilize the Immunological Garrison" was his phrase, and this motto dominated the work of one of the most advanced centers of medical research in Britain at that time.

It was in this department, in this atmosphere, that Alexander Fleming started his medical career. And it was in this department that he remained throughout his working life. Now it has been renamed: The Wright-Fleming Institute.

Chapter 3
FLEMING

AT THE GATE of a small farm, the last outpost of cultivation in Ayrshire in Southwest Scotland, there stands a simple, dignified monument erected by the local community. It is no more than a block of red granite bearing the words:

SIR ALEXANDER FLEMING
Discoverer of Penicillin
was born here at Lochfield
on 6th August, 1881

Perhaps it's partly the fault of Lochfield itself. It's not very romantic, simply the last farm before cultivation ceases, the borderline between the green and purple, soggy moorland of the southern Scottish uplands and the farms and woods that run down eventually to the Clyde coast. Not the dramatic mountain country of the real Highlands where there can be dreams and fairy tales, but a solid farm run by solid people where a real-life tale of the country-boy-made-good can start with the approval of all solid English-speaking people on both sides of the Atlantic. There is nature close by in the streams and moorlands; not nature "red-in-tooth-and-claw," but rabbits and little trout; there is a local country school (at least there was in the 1880s); a larger school in the country town of Darvel and an Academy at Kilmarnock where the sterling country lad could receive a basic education before he started for London. In London, in due course, working devotedly in his laboratory, that acute natural power of observation developed by his childhood play on the edge of the moors would enable him to perceive the importance of a chance occurrence which had probably been missed by others.

The truth of Fleming's childhood and youth is simple and undramatic. But throughout his life he was most determined to keep his private life separate from his professional activities, unknown if possible to his colleagues. So much so that it can fairly be said that he was secretive about his private life and affairs. The opposite side of the man is revealed by Dr. Howard Hughes, his assistant and professional colleague at the end of his working days:

> An opportunity to correct the impressions commonly held about Sir Alexander Fleming and his work is long overdue. He was himself responsible, to a large extent, for the misrepresentation which has arisen. It is well known that he was extremely shy and reticent about himself, it is less well recognized that he appeared to welcome the most unlikely reports on his discoveries since by them his personal privacy was maintained. During the later War years and immediately after, one of the duties of his secretary, Miss Pauline Hunter, was to collect and file reports and press cuttings connected with his work.
>
> One series we referred to as "The Fleming Myth"; in it were all the highly-coloured and often imaginary stories of the discovery of penicillin and of the man himself. These he never corrected, but rather treasured them as jokes to be recounted to his colleagues. As a consequence of his attitude, many of these stories have grown in the telling or on being passed from one journal to

another so that there is danger that the picture that he watched growing and that progressively approximates to "a barefooted peasant boy brought up on a scant diet of porridge with an occasional herring as a treat, educating himself, stumbling by accident on an important discovery that he neither worked for nor appreciated" will be taken as true. It is to be hoped that while some of those who worked with him are still alive the record can be put straight.

Alexander Fleming was born and brought up on a farm and received the training and education typical of the Lowland Scots of the Victorian period. He attended first the local school and then passed on to the grammar school serving the area. This background has produced many business and professional men and was an entirely adequate background for a university education. There were insufficient opportunities locally for the whole family, and while the farm provided a living for some, the others emigrated elsewhere. One brother worked in a shipping office in London, and he was joined by young Alexander. In his own private circle he was known as Sandy; a fact unknown to his later professional colleagues who called him either Alex or Flem.

So Fleming received the education which it was the particular pride of Scotland to provide for its country children, the education which launched so many Scottish younger sons into successful careers the world over at the turn of the century.

And it was a small legacy from an uncle that enabled him to leave the shipping office and study at the Polytechnic so successfully that he gained a scholarship in medicine to London University. Fleming then chose St. Mary's Hospital as the place where he would like to start as a medical student, and he made this choice, according to his own admission in later life, for little other reason than that he had swum and shot against student teams from St. Mary's when he had been representing a Territorial Army Unit in which he and his brother were keen "amateur soldiers."

Fleming started his medical studies in 1901. He performed brilliantly and qualified as a doctor on August 6, 1906, his twenty-fifth birthday. He immediately joined Sir Almroth Wright's Inoculation Department at St. Mary's and therefore he spent his entire professional life at that one hospital. The young Fleming had considered specializing in surgery, but he was well aware that one of the graduates of his year was likely to outshine him in this branch of medicine. He chose therefore to accept the honor of a research post in Wright's department not only on account of his examination successes, but also because Freeman, one of Wright's brilliant young assistants was interested in the hospital rifle-shooting team, and had heard that Fleming was a good shot. Fleming himself maintained in the days of his world renown that it was swimming and shooting that had made him a St. Mary's man and kept him one.

But the Inoculation Department, though it was humming with scientific life, a mecca for overseas visitors, especially postgraduate students, a new and exciting port of call for social and literary people, was very far from our present-day image of a research department. The physical conditions were atrocious. St. Mary's was by no means a fashionable hospital; it had been founded only during the nineteenth century, and therefore did not possess the endowments of the elder and more famous hospitals; its medical students tended to be men of much less wealth and social prestige than those at the more famous teaching schools. The hospital buildings were jammed in between Paddington railway station, the London terminus of the Great Western Railway, and the wharves of the Grand Union Canal. Much of the area served by the hospital consisted of poor quality housing, though there were also some very fashionable areas of large houses.

The teaching rooms of the Medical School were appallingly cold and dirty and most of the consultants and lecturers at the hospital only spent two half-days a week there, because they had to make their livings from treating private patients. Even in the 1920s very few of them had any time for research and the only laboratory available to the hospital was "a tiny room in the basement where the medical clerks tested urine." Against this background the Inoculation Department indeed seemed to be a place of cleanliness, scientific discipline, warmth and excitement. But it was in reality only four wards, each of which had originally been designed to hold six or seven patients, plus their ancillary offices, now converted into laboratories. It occupied four floors at the southeast corner of the hospital building, directly fronting onto Praed Street, which is the main road of approach to Paddington station. The architectural feature of the place was the almost circular turret going up the whole height of the building and containing on each floor a very small room. Immediately behind these turret rooms was a staircase and in the well of the staircase was an open elevator shaft. The entire elevator shaft was separated from the stairway by no more than a Victorian wrought-iron banister and thick, open-mesh wiring. It can all be seen very little changed to this day, with its half-tiled walls in those rather vivid lemon yellows and deep greens inexplicably favored by our ancestors.

From a working point of view these comparatively palatial laboratories of the Inoculation Department were already hopelessly overcrowded. Not even Sir Almroth Wright, the director, had a private room. Six or seven scientists might well be working in one room, giving each man no more than six feet of laboratory bench for his experiments and all his writing and paperwork.

> Privacy was completely unknown. . . . The room in which all the glassware was prepared and the media made was not much larger [than 15 feet square]. The darkroom had been converted from a very small w.c. and the hot room was a gas-operated death trap about the same size. Although the Department had appeared much more prosperous and better staffed than the Medical School, it was almost poverty-stricken by modern standards. We had to buy our own microscopes. There was no fume cupboard or sterile room. The nearest approach to a refrigerator was a wooden box about the size of a tea chest into which someone inserted a block of ice if he happened to remember. But one thing the place did possess, and that in abundance, was its smell: an all pervading odour of hot oil reminiscent of an engine room, which was produced by the heated oilbaths in which we sterilised our syringes.

Poverty-stricken, ill-equipped and smelly though it may have been, it was never, like the laboratories in the medical school, dirty and untidy. All the brassware—most of the apparatus was made of it—shone brightly; the white-tiled benches were cleaned every morning and there was always a cheerful fire in winter.

The memories are those of Professor Ronald Hare who joined the department shortly before Fleming's adventure with penicillin began. They therefore date from a full twenty years after Fleming himself first came, when, presumably, conditions were even more primitive.

In its early stages it was only Wright's personal generosity that kept the department going. He had crowded waiting rooms and many private patients from the wealthy and fashionable classes who called him in for any ailment from a boil to typhoid fever. And it was his fees from these patients that funded much of the research.

His young research workers therefore had to have private practices of their own as well. Wright made a virtue of this, declaring that it helped a man to "keep his feet on the ground." But it was also a necessity since he could not afford to pay his men more than £100 a year. Even by the 1920s salaries for beginners were only £300 a year. One serious disadvantage of this system was that it meant that salary levels and promotions for individuals depended on Wright's personal whims.

Some of the burden of supporting the department was taken away as it began to develop the commercial production of its own vaccines. This was on two levels. Some of the vaccines were developed by the department as a whole for sale to commercial pharmaceutical companies or other organizations. But each doctor also manufactured his own vaccines for sale to his own private patients. One who remembers those times says of Fleming: "He was always most meticulous about giving the department the time it paid him for. I remember he would never open the incubator and start handling his own private vaccine work until the clock had struck six."

Typical of the department's more commercial vaccine work was the Public Schools Vaccine scheme. The public schools of

Britain, as is widely known, are in fact private boarding schools, which, since they are fee-charging, are virtually the exclusive province of the rich and the wealthier middle class. Under the conditions of several hundred boys living the spartan life of an early-twentieth-century boarding school, epidemics of infectious disease could spread extremely rapidly. If the germ were virulent there could be deaths; an epidemic of diphtheria in a school was the setting of many a dramatic schoolboy story in my own youthful memories. If the germ was not so dangerous there could still be the virtual loss of a term's activities for many of the pupils. The Public Schools Vaccine scheme worked by taking swabs from all the boys when they assembled at the start of term. Appropriate vaccines would then be prepared against those germs most commonly found among the boys, and the entire school population would be vaccinated against the organisms that seemed to be most likely to cause trouble in that particular term. For an institution like the Inoculation Department such a scheme would provide a lot of their bread-and-butter, with which they could carry on their research, but it also meant a great deal of hard work preparing the inoculations. Work well into the small hours of the morning was not merely commonplace, it was the norm at the time Fleming joined the department.

Fleming's early work was performed under Wright's immediate direction and consisted largely of building up the technique that demonstrated the opsonic index and enabled it to be used. These were almost all small-scale techniques; they were, for those days, advanced micro-techniques. They involved mostly laboratory glassware and the use of the microscope. And Fleming quickly showed that he was a real master of this sort of craft. All those who remember him at work are agreed that he could perform miracles with the most elementary laboratory glassware. Wright acknowledged Fleming's work majestically in one paper "My colleague Dr. Alexander Fleming has given in the treatise which is prefaced by these remarks of mine an admirable summing up of the results obtained by the Inoculation Department at St. Mary's Hospital. . . ." From a man who once took up three full issues of the *Lancet* with one paper, a man who all too often added his own name to the papers describing work done by his assistants, this was both a stamp of approval and an admission that most of the results which followed were Fleming's.

It was almost certainly this acknowledged manual dexterity and his reputation for surgical promise (he had obtained his Fellowship of the Royal College of Surgeons before deciding in favor of bacteriology) that gained for Fleming a most important opportunity. One of Wright's friends was that stupendous figure of the German scientific effort, Paul Ehrlich. Ehrlich was basically a chemist who became one of the great pioneers of immunology, and yet produced the world's first successful chemotherapeutic drug. As a student Ehrlich had been fascinated by the scientific developments which were really a consequence of the first rise of the German chemical-dye industry. With the new chemical dyes it was possible to stain micro-organisms and the tissues of larger creatures, not only so that they became visible under the microscope, but also in a specific manner. It has already been mentioned that some bacteria were stained by Gram's stain and so are still called Gram-positive, while others do not take up this stain. A more apposite example in this context is that methylene blue is specific or selective in staining nerve tissue, and this enabled the German microscopists to follow the course of the nerves through masses of other tissue. It had also been shown that the toxins of certain bacteria (diphtheria and tetanus particularly) attacked specific parts of the body such as the heart muscles or the nerve cells.

From this Ehrlich started his search for what he called "the magic bullet." This was the chemical that would specifically attack one particular type of microbe in the same way that a stain would attach itself to one particular type of microbe. In due course the dye chemists came up with a substance, a compound of arsenic called atoxyl, which was shown to kill trypanosomes and spirochetes. These are organisms rather more complex than bacteria, which cause diseases of men and animals. In particular one variety of spirochete causes syphilis. Atoxyl, which was produced between 1905 and 1907, was unfortunately highly toxic to animals as well as to micro-organisms, but nevertheless Ehrlich started a grinding and thorough campaign to produce new arsenical compounds, variants on the atoxyl molecule, and to screen them one by one for activity against micro-organisms and for non-toxicity to animals. The 606th such compound synthesized in 1909 proved to be a destroyer of spirochetes without killing the test mice and guinea pigs. And in the summer of 1909 it was shown to have remarkable curative powers when treating syphilitic lesions in rabbits. This was Salvarsan or Arsphenamine, the first chemotherapeutic ever to be found by science, the first chemical that could be used in the living body to destroy micro-organisms. (Quinine, which has been used for centuries in the treatment of malaria, was discovered empirically in South America and was in one sense the first chemotherapeutic agent if we discount the ancient herbal remedies.)

Ehrlich brought some samples of Salvarsan when he visited London in 1910 and gave them to his friend Wright. Because it was so difficult to handle, Fleming was deputed to treat patients with it. Salvarsan arrived as a powder which had to be dissolved in water at the bedside of the patient who was to be treated. It had to be injected intravenously—that is to say, right into a blood vessel—and if too much escaped into the surrounding tissue it could result in the loss of the entire arm. It was so dangerous that only one dose could be given every seven days, but even so treatment might go on for a year before the syphilis was finally cleared up.

Thus Fleming became probably the first doctor in Britain to use Salvarsan. And there arose a number of delicious ironies. The institution which was the fountainhead of the doctrine that "Drugs are a delusion" was the leading user of the first effective drug against micro-organisms, yet the doctrine was preached with ever greater vigor.

And Fleming himself became "one of the leading venereologists in London before the war." The mythical picture of the dedicated research worker toiling alone in his laboratory just could not have been true in the Britain of those days. To us in the 1970s being a research worker is a fulltime and reasonably well-paid occupation; we recognize that research is a worthwhile investment for society as a whole and for groupings within society such as industrial concerns. These are axioms to us; they were not accepted in the first decade of our century, and a research worker like Fleming had to earn his living in private practice.

Furthermore, this activity of Fleming's may well have some bearing on the development of the penicillin story. For the rest of his life Fleming was financially comfortable, though he was never a rich man; though he gave his later awards to research and though he died worth little more than the value of the cash prize that went with his Nobel award. But he had his comfortable country home in Suffolk which he visited almost every weekend for many years, as well as his London home, which was a Chelsea flat. In other words he was not pressed for money in his middle life and this may have blunted the cutting edge of his aggression and personal ambition in the pursuit of penicillin.

It is likely that his private practice brought him into touch with artists, and this would account for his years of membership of the Chelsea Arts Club. Throughout the 1920s and 1930s and well on into his later years he was a most regular member of this club. A drink and a game of snooker in the evening was his most frequent relaxation there, and yet he was in no way artistic. It is an otherwise almost inexplicable anomaly in his pattern of life.

But the first major event in his life was World War I, when he went with most of Wright's group to work in a special research laboratory in the Casino at Boulogne where they struggled with the problems of battle injuries and specifically with the difficulties of septic wounds. Septicemia, gangrene and tetanus were the most feared complications of injuries caused by high explosives, bullets or shrapnel in the filthy conditions of the trenches, where earth or scraps of dirty clothing almost inevitably got into the damaged tissues.

It was in these surroundings that Fleming did what many

people (notably Freeman) regard as the best scientific work of his life. Stemming from Pasteur's original germ work, and parallel with the development of immunology, there had developed aseptic surgery. Lister had been the prime mover in this development and his ideas of passing everything in the operating theater, from smocks to scalpels, through antiseptic solutions, had won fairly rapid acceptance. Some sterilizing was done by heat in autoclaves, but a number of fairly powerful antiseptics other than Lister's carbolic had been discovered. Surgeons had learned how to stop germs getting into the incisions they made, and surgery had been revolutionized as a result. But the antiseptic treatment of surgical instruments to prevent wounds being infected was a very different matter from the antiseptic treatment of wounds already infected. Packing wounds with antiseptics such as boric acid, hydrogen peroxide and the old favorite, carbolic, was standard medical practice; since a high proportion of the medical establishment were pupils and disciples of Lister, it was likely to remain so.

Fleming's war work showed quite clearly that in infected wounds the phagocytes of the body's normal defenses were both more numerous and more active than in clean wounds. And furthermore he showed that the standard antiseptics killed all white cells faster and more effectively than they killed microbes. He supported this with evidence that antiseptics in wounds not only failed to prevent gangrene, but actually seemed to increase its speed of development. In other words, antiseptics in already infected wounds made things worse instead of better by doing more damage to the natural defenses than to the microbes. Finally, by one of his best tricks with laboratory glassware, Fleming created a rough model of the ragged and torn tissues of a wound (the anfractuosities in the medical parlance of the day) in the bottom of a test-tube, and then allowed bacteria to spread into the indentations and roughnesses of the glass. Washing after washing with antiseptics of all sorts and strengths failed to dislodge the microorganisms and Fleming could show a reinfection of fresh, clean, uninfected, human blood serum every time he allowed it into contact with the glass wound.

In practical terms this demolition of one theory did not lead to much advance. Fleming and Wright saw that the best way of improving the chances of wound healing was to persuade the surgeons to cut away as much damaged and dying tissue as possible. They tried to improve the supply of phagocytes to the wound by bathing with strong saline solution, and toward the end of the war by giving blood transfusions. For the wounded soldiers there was not much advance, it is true; for Wright it meant opportunities for further enormous disputes with the army medical authorities. He involved his personal friends in the cabinet in these rows; and he fought a drawn battle in bitter public controversy with Sir William Watson Cheyne, the president of the Royal College of Surgeons. George Bernard Shaw, a frequent visitor to the Boulogne laboratories, became a keen observer and backroom participant in the uproar. For Fleming, it is clear that the work simply strengthened the case against chemotherapy and must have helped to keep his mind closed to the true potentialities of penicillin when he came across it in due course.

There were, in fact, a whole series of new antiseptics developed in the first twenty-five years of this century. Each one had great claims made for it, and each one turned out to be equally useless at killing germs inside the body, whatever it might have done to microbes in the laboratory test tubes and culture plates.

There was mercurochrome, a compound of mercury much favored in the U.S.A., and sponsored there by many distinguished clinicians. It was given to Balfour (then Lord Balfour) on a visit to America when he developed a sore throat. He gargled with mercurochrome and the sore throat disappeared. Since he was Lord President of the Council (an ancient British title mostly meaningless nowadays, it's often given to a cabinet minister whose responsibilities are a rag-bag of affairs not covered by the usual ministries) and responsible to Parliament for the Medical Research Council, on his return he requested the secretary of the council, Sir Walter Morley Fletcher, to start research into this wonder drug. In due course the work devolved on Dr. Leonard Colebrook in Wright's department

and from him to Ronald Hare. It was soon shown that mercurochrome was "singularly ineffective even in the test-tube,
and still more so in the tissues."

Colebrook and Hare, again with Medical Research Council
support, and after they had left St. Mary's, were among those
who pursued the line of the arsenicals, hoping that Salvarsan
would have useful chemical relatives. There was no progress.
Then there was Sanocrysin, the gold treatment for tuberculosis, invented in Denmark and much in vogue in the 1920s. It
was Almroth Wright himself who showed that doses twenty
times as large as those that any doctor dared give to a human
patient left the tubercle bacilli growing unchecked in the test-
tube.

Clinicians in general became deeply suspicious of any new
claim for an antiseptic, or indeed for any chemical treatment;
there had been too many false alarms. Fleming mentioned the
almost mystical belief that once the microbes had got inside
the body they could never be attacked. And Fleming contributed to the list of failed antiseptics with his discovery of
lysozyme. The discovery was by any standards a major contribution to knowledge, for lysozyme, which Fleming discovered
to be present in tears, turned out to be a constituent of most
of the mucous fluids of human and animal bodies and to be a
major component of egg albumen. Most of this was established by Fleming himself, and late in his life he still held that
lysozyme could be more important than penicillin.

The account of the discovery of lysozyme is related in the
Maurois biography of Fleming entirely in the words of Dr.
V.D. Allison, who was at that time, 1922, a newly appointed
assistant. Fleming was cleaning up some Petri dishes:

> As he took up one of the dishes in his hand he looked at it for a
> long time, showed it to me and said "This is interesting." I had
> a good look at it. It was covered with large yellow colonies which
> appeared to me to be obvious contaminants. But the remarkable
> fact was that there was a wide area in which there were no or-
> ganisms; and another further one in which the organisms had

become translucent and glassy. Beyond that again were organisms which were in a transitional stage of degradation, between the very glassy ones and those which were fully developed with their normal pigment.

Fleming explained that this particular dish was one to which he had added a little of his own nasal mucus, when he had happened to have a cold. This mucus was in the middle of the zone containing no colony. The idea at once occurred to him that there must be something in the mucus which dissolved or killed the microbes in its immediate neighbourhood and then became diffused in such a way that it progressively contaminated the already developed colonies. "Now that really is interesting," he said again. "We must go into it more thoroughly." His first care was to pick off the organism and stain it by Gram. He found it was a large Gram-positive coccus, not a pathogen, and not one of the known saprophytic organisms commonly met with, but obviously a contaminating organism which was more likely to have been in the atmosphere of the laboratory, and may, of course, have blown in through the window from the dust and air of Praed Street.

The story of the discovery of lysozyme is so extraordinarily similar to the penicillin story in its little externals—the remarks made, the action taken, the contaminant from Praed Street—that any historian is entitled to surmise that in the years between the 1920s when these things happened and the 1940s and 1950s when they were told, the myth of penicillin had already started to form among Fleming's colleagues. But the essentials are almost exactly the opposite of the penicillin observation. For lysozyme, the antibacterial, came from the laboratory and it was the contaminant organism that was destroyed. And in lysozyme the disappointment came from the fact that the rare contaminant was the one bacterium in the world that is most easily destroyed by lysozyme. It was a bacterium previously unknown to science, quite harmless to man, which Fleming had the privilege of naming *Micrococcus lysodeikticus,* the organism which demonstrates the power of dissolving.

The disappointment of finding that lysozyme was much

less effective against dangerous, pathogenic germs did not stop Fleming from pursuing the creature itself. He correctly showed that lysozyme was an enzyme, one of the group of substances which cause or catalyze the innumerable complicated chemical reactions which go on within living bodies. He showed that it is to be found widely distributed throughout the plant and animal kingdoms. The very fact that it was not particularly effective against disease-causing germs fitted into Fleming's final theory (which we believe to be perfectly correct) that lysozyme is one of the great natural protective substances. In the human being and animal it is the first line of defense, long before the immune system comes into operation, and lysozyme is found particularly in those exposed areas, such as the eye and the mucus of the nose where there is no blood supply and therefore the immune system cannot operate.

We can never know how much the discovery of lysozyme misled Fleming when it came to the time of penicillin six years afterward, but there is plenty to imply that it played an important part, particularly from the nature of the way in which it was discovered. But the ineffectiveness of lysozyme as an antibacterial must have closed Fleming's mind even more firmly toward the possibility of effective chemotherapy. And the cold reaction of the medical and scientific world to the announcements of his discovery must have been in many ways even more frustrating.

The medical world of the time is less to be blamed for its attitude than Fleming's partisans make out; not only was Fleming an extremely poor speaker and lecturer, but the important paper in which he first announced the discovery of lysozyme quite literally *does not make sense*. The paper, published in the great prestige of the *Proceedings of the Royal Society* and "Communicated by Sir Almroth Wright, F.R.S." is titled "On a remarkable Bacteriolytic element found in tissues and secretions." Its opening paragraphs read:

> In this communication I wish to draw attention to a substance present in the tissues and secretions of the body, which is capable

of rapidly dissolving certain bacteria. As this substance has properties akin to those of ferments [i.e. what we now call enzymes] I have called it a "Lysozyme," and shall refer to it by this name throughout the communication.

The lysozyme was first noticed during some investigations made on a patient suffering from acute coryza. [Coryza means common cold and the patient was, of course, Fleming himself.] The nasal secretion of this patient was cultivated daily on blood-agar plates, and for the first three days of the infection there was no growth with the exception of an occasional staphylococcus colony. The culture made from the nasal mucus on the fourth day showed in twenty-four hours a large number of small colonies which, on examination, proved to be large Gram-positive cocci arranged irregularly but with a tendency to diplococcal and tetrad formation. It is necessary to give here a very brief description of this microbe as with it most of the experiments described below were done, and it was with it that the phenomena to be described were best manifested. The microbe has not been exactly identified, but for purposes of this communication it may be alluded to as the *Micrococcus lysodeikticus*.

He then goes on to note the observations he made on the microbe, and immediately goes into a section titled "Preliminary experiments showing the action of the lysozyme."

On the face of it each of the sentences of the first two paragraphs is grammatical and makes sense. But a second reading shows that having said "the lysozyme was first noticed" he does not report how or why the lysozyme was noticed or that there was any clue to its ability to destroy the microbe. It appears in fact that one or two complete sentences must have been left out.

When it came to writing Fleming's official "scientific" biography, which is done for all Fellows of the Royal Society in the form of *Memoirs*, the loyal former colleague, Leonard Colebrook, duly noted the double nature of the discovery: the finding of the lysozyme itself and the finding of the microbe which was particularly susceptible to it. He then quotes from the first two paragraphs of the paper and is reduced by its incomprehensibility to putting in a footnote which reads "Dr. V.D. Allison, who collaborated with Fleming in much of his lysozyme work, tells me that Fleming thought these micrococci did not actually come from his nose, but were chance contaminants blown onto the plate from the air."

And the official *Memoir* continues: "It is not quite clear what led Fleming to suspect that there was something in the nasal mucus which would exert a powerful lytic action on this microbe. Probably there were some areas on his plate cultures where the growth of the micrococcus was inhibited or prevented by particles of mucus. At any rate he did suspect it and his suspicions were confirmed."

The significance of this matter is not that it throws any sinister light on Fleming but that it reveals what was his greatest weakness: his quite extraordinary inability to communicate. Whatever may have been the factors which later held him back from pursuing penicillin more aggressively, he would certainly fail to communicate his original interest and excitement, the interest which his genuine results should have aroused, to others.

Among those who still remember Fleming one remarked, "He had an almost pathological inability to communicate." Professor Chain's memory of Fleming's first visit to Oxford many years later to see Chain's penicillin was that Fleming did not say a word about it. Even Colebrook's official *Memoir* mentions this aspect of the man: "Fleming was a man of few words —and ideas did not greatly interest him. Women on meeting him for the first time were often nonplussed by the unemotional, 'almost basilisk' stare, which some of them mistook for rudeness, while others were fascinated. But there was much friendliness and kindness behind that apparently cold exterior, as many can testify."

Perhaps even more vivid, because more personal, are a few sentences from Professor Hare. Writing about the pleasant gossiping in the Inoculation Department he says:

> Fleming was no exception, and in order to do so had to leave his little room down the staircase to find someone with whom to gossip. He had, therefore, evolved the custom of indulging in a

morning potter, which included a visit to the big laboratory in which I was working.

Fleming's idea of gossip was different from that of most other people. It usually involved his planting himself in front of the fireplace, with his hands in his pockets, a cigarette dangling from his lips, and looking more or less into space. On rare occasions he would give utterance, usually in the fewest possible words. The information doled out so meagrely might concern anything; that so-and-so had died; that what's-his-name had made a fool of himself again; or how are your Snia Viscosas doing [Snia Viscosa was the name of a stock-market share]?

Fleming was a man very much loved by the many who knew him well, by those who passed beyond the barriers of his silences. There is no doubt too that the concealed man had a fine character, just, honest, generous and loving. But it is an essential part of the scientist's work to communicate properly, at least with his fellow scientists. His inability in this field was Fleming's greatest professional weakness.

Strangely enough Fleming was not shy of broadcasting or meeting journalists and writers. David Masters describes how he was made welcome to his laboratory in the days of his fame in 1945, and Fleming went to great trouble to demonstrate the action of lysozyme and show how it had first been discovered. The fact that he chose, even then when penicillin had made him famous, to demonstrate the early work on lysozyme and not to show how penicillin had been found, can now be seen to be highly significant.

Chapter 4
FLEMING AND PENICILLIN

By 1928 THE SITUATION in the Inoculation Department at St. Mary's Hospital had changed greatly. Fleming had been appointed professor of bacteriology and deputy director of the department. New buildings were being erected to house the department, buildings which now form the core of the Wright-Fleming Institute of St. Mary's Hospital Medical School. The administrative load on Fleming had increased materially.

Sir Almroth Wright was over sixty years old, growing slightly more mellow and a little more tolerant of his juniors doing work of which he disapproved. But still he dominated them all and still the flow of magisterial talk continued. The greatest problem was in the relationship between Wright and Dr. J.B. Freeman, the man Wright had once called his "son in science." Freeman was as different from Fleming as it was possible to be; he was blond, good-looking, cultivated, with an Oxford background, and a superb conversationalist who accompanied Wright when the tea-time talk soared up into the imaginative stratosphere. He felt that Wright had promised him the succession to the headship of the department, and had gone back on his promise by appointing Fleming as professor. However, Freeman never quarreled with Fleming personally. His real dispute with Wright concerned Wright's insistence on putting his own name on Freeman's most important scientific publication.

Freeman had turned to the study of allergy, which had been known to be an immunological subject for many years. He established the view that hay fever is an allergy to windborne pollen, a view that holds the field to the present day. But Wright had insisted on putting his own name on Freeman's first important paper on the matter, although he had neither advised upon, nor directed, the work. The practice of a senior professor putting his name first on a paper describing a junior colleague's work is by no means unknown today, but it is felt in many scientific centers to smack too much of the old Germanic idea of the professor dominating a department which is his own personal kingdom. The defense of the practice is that the professor, by lending the weight and fame of his name, draws attention to the younger man's work.

The result of these frictions was to split the department into at least two main, and separate groups of workers. Young newcomers were appointed either to Fleming's side or to Freeman's without regard to their desires or qualifications, but simply in order to keep the two sides equal. Dr. Howard Hughes suggests that one reason for lack of interest in Fleming's observation of penicillin was the enervating effect of these internal rivalries; there were many in the department who treated the discovery of penicillin as just another of the rather pointless natural observations that Fleming was prone to making. Undoubtedly, also, the medical world outside St. Mary's had come to dislike the pugnacious and argumentative attitude of Sir Almroth Wright, and tended to deride any announcements that came from him or his colleagues.

There is no shred of evidence that Wright in any way attempted to stifle or hold back Fleming's work on penicillin, which pointed so strongly toward the development of chemotherapy: the use of drugs to cure disease or infection. But Wright did not believe that chemotherapy offered any solution to medical problems; nor did Fleming. Indeed, his best and most fruitful scientific work, in the Boulogne studies of war wounds, had provided the strongest evidence backing this viewpoint. It would be asking a very great deal of human nature to expect these men to have abandoned the strongly held well-backed views of their scientific maturity, and to have hurled themselves wholeheartedly into the support and follow-up of Fleming's strange observation.

So it was in a very unpromising intellectual milieu that penicillin made its first scientific appearance. Many accounts of this occasion have been published. Most of them come originally from the small spate of books written about penicillin in the late 1940s and early 1950s. Fleming was never pompous, stuffy or shy. He was easily available to journalists and writers; he always entertained them kindly when they came seeking his reminiscences and he could quite easily be persuaded to give enthusiastic "lab demonstrations" of various aspects of his work. He also broadcast on the radio quite willingly and even made a number of television appearances. Broadly speaking, all this material originated roughly twenty years after the first observation of penicillin, but despite this gap in years the stories are remarkably consistent in their main features and there are only a small number of comparatively minor discrepancies between the various accounts of the historic moment of discovery.

There is, however, absolutely no knowledge about the exact date on which Fleming made his original observation. Fleming could not remember, and there seems to be no written record. The most usual version among the early accounts is that it was on a Monday late in August or early in September 1928, and that it occurred as Fleming was looking through a pile of his laboratory dishes on his return from a week's holiday at his country house.

What may be described as the official version of the moment of discovery comes in the Maurois biography of Fleming, which the famous French author wrote at the request of the second Lady Fleming. This does not even subscribe to the "return from holiday" story, but simply tells how, in 1928, Fleming was studying staphylococci in order to prepare a Medical Research Council publication article on bacteriology. He had established a large number of cultures of the organism on substrates of agar in glass Petri dishes. On the crucial day he was visited by Merlyn Pryce, formerly his assistant, who had himself done important research on staphylococci.

> Pryce went to see Fleming in his little laboratory, where he found him, as usual, surrounded by innumerable dishes. The cautious Scot disliked being separated from his cultures before he was quite certain that there was no longer anything to be learned from them. He was often teased about his disorderly habits. He was now to prove that disorder may have its uses. With his rough humour he reproached Pryce for obliging him to re-do a long job of work, and, while speaking took up several old cultures and removed the lids. Several of the cultures had been contaminated by mould—a not unusual occurrence. "As soon as you uncover a culture dish something tiresome is sure to happen. Things fall out of the air." Suddenly he stopped talking, then, after a moment's observation, said in his usual unconcerned tones: "That's funny . . ." On the culture at which he was looking there was a growth of mould, as on several of the others, but on this particular one, all round the mould, the colonies of staphylococci had been dissolved and, instead of forming opaque yellow masses, looked like drops of dew.
>
> Pryce had often seen old microbial colonies which for various reasons had dissolved. He thought that probably the mould was producing acids which were harmful to the staphylococci—no unusual occurrence. But, noticing the keen interest with which Fleming was examining the phenomenon, he said: "That's how you discovered lysozyme." Fleming made no answer. He was busy taking a little piece of the mould with his scalpel and putting it in a tube of broth. Then he picked off a scrap measuring about one square millimetre which floated on the surface of the broth.

He obviously wanted to make quite sure that this mysterious mould would be preserved.

There is unfortunately an aura of hagiography about this otherwise well-told story. It lacks detail in describing what it was that so much interested Fleming in the contaminated plate; that differentiated it from other contaminated plates; that others did not note. By examining his later, more scientific, descriptions and by studying the photos of the original plate we can see: the well-developed mold growth on one side of the plate was surrounded firstly by an area in which there were no staphylococci at all; then by another band in which there appeared to be "ghost" or destroyed colonies of staphylococci; the colonies of staphylococci were progressively better defined as one moved across this zone away from the mold; the remainder of the dish contained perfectly healthy, well-grown colonies of normal staphylococci. It seemed to Fleming that it was likely that a substance produced by the mold had diffused through the agar-jelly substrate and had progressively destroyed colonies of staphylococci as it had spread out.

But let us be good historians and go back to the original source, the official scientific publication of Fleming's observation. This is his historic paper "On the antibacterial action of cultures of a penicillium with special reference to their use in the isolation of *B. influenzae*," which was published in the *British Journal of Experimental Pathology*. It is marked "Received for publication May 10th, 1929." The first paragraph reads: "While working with staphylococcus variants a number of culture plates were set aside on the laboratory bench and examined from time to time. In the examinations these plates were necessarily exposed to the air and they became contaminated with various micro-organisms. It was noticed that around a large colony of a contaminating mould the staphylococcus colonies became transparent and were obviously undergoing lysis." And he includes a photograph of the famous plate.

This paragraph tells very little and it has been criticized by well-qualified scientists for its inadequacies. It does not say which varieties of staphylococcus were being used; nor does it say what was the medium on which they were being grown. It does not say whether the plates had been incubated or at what temperatures they had been kept. It does not say how old the plates were, how big the mold colony was, how many colonies of staphylococci were alive and well, how many were undergoing lysis or at what range from the mold the changes were taking place. These omissions turned out to be of great importance later.

The paper goes on to describe how Fleming immediately set about subculturing the mold which seemed to have produced the effect, and this single action was probably his most important contribution to the development of penicillin. He grew the mold in various nutrient solutions and at various different temperatures; he tested its products for acidity and alkalinity. He wrote it all up in the rather friendly style which was then customary even in an academic, scientific publication:

> The colony appears as a white fluffy mass which rapidly increases in size and after a few days sporulates, the centre becoming dark green and later in old cultures darkens almost to black. In four or five days a bright yellow colour is produced which diffuses into the medium. In certain conditions a reddish colour can be observed in the growth.
>
> In broth the mould grows on the surface as a white fluffy growth changing in a few days to a dark green felted mass. The broth becomes bright yellow and this yellow pigment is not extracted by $CHCl_3$. The reaction of the broth becomes markedly alkaline, the pH varying from 8.5 to 9. Acid is produced in three or four days in glucose and saccharose broth. There is no acid production in seven days in lactose, mannite or dulcite broth. Growth is slow at 37°C and is most rapid about 20°C. No growth is observed under anaerobic conditions.

With the benefit of hindsight many significant phrases can be picked out of this short extract. "The mould grows on the surface" is one such phrase. The different rates of growth on different media and at different temperatures also become significant in the story later on. There is also the mention of acidity and alkalinity in which lay the eventual clues to the extraction of penicillin.

Fleming's next task was to see whether the production of antibacterial substances was common to molds of many kinds. He examined five other species of molds and eight different types of penicillium molds. He does not say in his paper where he got these molds or why he chose these particular ones. But in the acknowledgments at the end of the paper he thanks "our mycologist Mr. La Touche" (C.J. La Touche) for his suggestions as to the identity of the penicillium. La Touche, the mycologist of the department, almost certainly played a larger part in the discovery of penicillin than he has usually been given credit for, even if the part played was involuntary. He identified the mold on Fleming's original plate as a penicillium, most likely *Penicillium rubrum*. In this he was wrong, it was a *Penicillium notatum*. He subsequently apologized to Fleming for this mistaken identification and accepted full responsibility for his mistake. It made no difference at all, even when the proper identity of Fleming's mold was established years later by the American mycologist, Dr. Charles Thom. Poor La Touche is one of those who have gone into history for the wrong reason.

The molds that Fleming tried out were *Eidamia viridescens*, *Botrytis cineria*, *Aspergillus fumigatus*, *Sporotrichum*, *Cladosporium*, and the eight strains of penicillium. The remark he makes on this is of enormous significance: "Of these it was found that only one strain of penicillium produced any inhibitory substance, and that one had exactly the same cultural characters as the original one from the contaminated plate." In terms of science this meant that Fleming's observation had indeed been an important one. He had truly observed an unusual phenomenon produced by a particular species of mold, a specific action and not a generalized interaction. He wrote: "It is clear, therefore, that the production of this antibacterial substance is not common to all moulds or to all types of penicillium."

But what was the origin of the one strain of penicillium which did produce the inhibitory substance and which appeared identical with the original? It is indeed most extraordinary that Fleming should not even mention this. In describing the mold and its behavior Fleming had shown one of his facets: the keen natural observer delighting in perhaps rather irrelevant colors and general appearances. In the next section of the paper he shows himself as the experienced bacteriologist and here he is at his scientific best, with, incidentally, his communication unusually clear, telling exactly what he did:

> The simplest method of examining for inhibitory power is to cut a furrow in an agar plate (or a plate of other suitable culture material), and fill this in with a mixture of equal parts of agar and the broth in which the mould has grown. When this has solidified, cultures of various microbes can be streaked at right angles from the furrow to the edge of the plate. The inhibitory substance diffuses very rapidly in the agar, so that in the few hours before the microbes show visible growth it has spread out for a centimetre or more in sufficient concentration to inhibit growth of a sensitive microbe. On further incubation it will be seen that the proximal portion of the culture for perhaps one centimetre becomes transparent and on examination of this portion of the culture it is found that practically all the microbes are dissolved, indicating that the antibacterial substance has continued to diffuse into the agar in sufficient concentration to induce dissolution of the bacteria. This simple method therefore suffices to demonstrate the bacterio-inhibitory and bacteriolytic properties of the mould culture, and also, by the extent of the area of inhibition gives some measure of the sensitiveness of the particular microbe tested.

Using this method, he successfully and correctly demonstrated that the substance produced by his mold would inhibit and destroy staphylococci, streptococci, the gonococci which cause gonorrhea, the meningococci (the organisms causing meningitis), the diphtheria bacillus, the pneumococcus and a number of bacteria which are not normally harmful to man. He had likewise shown that his "mold broth filtrate" was powerless against the agents of typhoid and cholera, and many of the other bacteria of the intestines. *B. pyocyaneus* and *B. proteus,* common causes of wound infection, were similarly unaffected, and, perhaps unfortunately as it turned out, *B. influenzae*, the Pfeiffer bacillus, which was at that time suspected of causing influenza, was also unharmed by the filtrate. A broad distinction seemed to be that those bacteria called Gram-positive were susceptible to the filtrate, while those called Gram-negative were resistant to it.

More than this, Fleming correctly found that there were some strains of streptococci which were unaffected by the bacterio-inhibitory substance. (In his later work he was almost certainly the first to recognize and isolate a genuine penicillin-resistant strain of bacteria.)

Two other important achievements were recorded by Fleming in his first paper. Using the staphylococci which had first revealed the presence of an unusual substance by their death (at least we presume he used the same variety, he does not actually say so) as a rough standard of the killing power of his mold-broth filtrate, he established that when the mold was started growing on a new plate it took five days before it started producing the antibacterial substance. On the fifth day one drop of the broth containing the substance diluted in twenty drops of distilled water killed the test bacteria. By the eighth day of culture the broth was at its maximum potency, and then one drop of broth diluted in 500 drops of water was sufficient to kill. In other words the potency of his substance was measurable and it was a very powerful substance indeed. Eventually he was able to find, under the right circumstances, broths which would kill staphylococci at a dilution of 1:600.

Finally, though he did not know it at the time, Fleming showed the one quality that really made his observation supremely important. He showed that it was not toxic. It is easy enough to find a chemical that kills bacteria. It is rare indeed to find a substance which is more dangerous to bacteria than to other creatures such as animals and men which are normally the hosts to the bacteria. Fleming recorded this non-toxicity soberly, almost in an aside:

The toxicity to animals of powerfully antibacterial mould-broth filtrates appears to be very low. Twenty cubic centimetres injected intravenously into a rabbit were not more toxic than the same quantity of broth. Half a cubic centimetre injected intraperitoneally into a mouse weighing about twenty grams induced no toxic symptoms. Constant irrigation of large infected surfaces in man was not accompanied by any toxic symptoms, while irrigation of the human conjunctiva every hour for a day had no irritant effect.

In vitro penicillin which completely inhibits the growth of staphylococci in a dilution of 1:600 does not interfere with leucocytic function to a greater extent than does ordinary broth.

This is Fleming at his most "dead pan." Take that last sentence: leucocytic function means the action of the human body's leucocytes or white cells, the functioning of the body's normal defense mechanisms. Yet it was Fleming who had demonstrated and preached the doctrine that all the antiseptics discovered up to that time killed off the leucocytes quicker than they killed invading bacteria. This had been the essence of his war-time work and it was the basis of his theoretical opposition to chemotherapy.

And those injections into rabbit and mouse are enormous: half a cubic centimeter into a twenty-gram mouse may not sound like much, but it means approximately one fortieth of its body weight, about the same as injecting four pounds of material into a 160-pound man. If that amount of the mold-broth filtrate was not poisonous, then it really was a safe substance.

Notice, too, that the substance had already been used in human ailments, but that Fleming does not even bother to mention whether it did any good to the sufferers. It is in this first paper, also, that we have the naming of penicillin. In one of the earliest paragraphs he coins the word that was to become known the world over.

There are, however, the negative aspects of his observation, and Fleming, always honest and objective in scientific matters, duly noted them. "Penicillin loses most of its power after ten or fourteen days at room temperature, but can be preserved longer by neutralization." That was the fourth, and in practical terms the most depressing, of the ten conclusions he drew. And in the fifth conclusion he pointed out that the power of penicillin rapidly disappeared when it was heated. It also appeared to be insoluble in ether or chloroform (which is not at all the irrelevancy it appears to modern eyes, for it predicted the terrible difficulties which would be found by everyone in isolating the active antibacterial substance).

Here, in brief, Fleming presented all the problems of penicillin which in actual fact prevented his observation and his first work from being the breakthrough which it is so often—wrongly—called. The stuff, whatever it was, in his mold-broth filtrate, was unmanageable. It could not be isolated in any of the readily available and usual chemical ways. It was highly unstable and simply disappeared, not only when he tried to manipulate it or concentrate it in any way, but even if he just left it standing about. It was therefore virtually useless from a clinical point of view. It took eight days to grow the mold on the fluid until there was a high concentration of power in the broth, and then ten or fourteen days later there was nothing left. This meant that unless the needs of the patient happened to coincide, in time, with the preparation of a laboratory brew there was no chance of trying it out.

The last two paragraphs of the paper show Fleming not at his best. They read:

> Penicillin, in regard to infections with sensitive microbes, appears to have some advantages over the well-known chemical antiseptics. A good sample will completely inhibit staphylococci, *Streptococcus pyogenes* and pneumococcus in a dilution of 1:800. It is therefore a more powerful inhibitory agent than is carbolic acid, and it can be applied to an infected surface undiluted as it is non-irritant and non-toxic. If applied, therefore, on a dressing it will still be effective even when diluted 800 times which is more than can be said of the chemical antiseptics in use. Experiments in connection with its value in the treatment of pyogenic infections are in progress.

In addition to its possible use in the treatment of bacterial infections penicillin is certainly useful to the bacteriologist for its power of inhibiting unwanted microbes in bacterial cultures so that penicillin-insensitive bacteria can be readily isolated. A notable instance of this is the very easy isolation of Pfeiffer's bacillus of influenza when penicillin is used.

The first sentences are repetitious and not entirely logical. Then there is the sentence about experiments in the treatment of infections. No details are given here, nor did Fleming in his later papers ever refer to these experiments. The biography and the early versions of the Fleming story cast no light, and there is no relevant reminiscence by any of those who worked with Fleming. The sentence remains a mystery.

Then there is the final paragraph which refers back to the title of the paper "with special reference to their use in the isolation of *B. influenzae,*" and also refers to a long section within the paper giving details of the work. This, in fact, is what Fleming used his penicillin for, and this is, for practical purposes, all that penicillin was ever used for during the next twelve years.

The logic of it is obvious and presumably represents something close to Fleming's thought process. The original contaminant had removed certain bacteria from a culture. This fortunate observation could be used to keep further cultures free of contamination.

Since penicillin was selective and killed only certain bacteria, this selective power could be used to isolate certain insensitive bacteria from the messy, mixed-up collections of bacteria that come in clinical situations when you actually examine or take swabs from human noses or throats. Fleming was interested in the influenza bacillus and he later became interested in the organism that causes whooping cough. He was interested, too, in the whole of the area of research known as bacterial antagonism, where the presence of one bacteria prevents the development of a different type of bacteria. He came to regard his penicillin as an extremely useful laboratory tool for his own work as a practicing bacteriologist. And it is a fact that, for the next ten years at least, it was a regular weekly chore for his research assistants and technicians to make a brew of penicillin for this laboratory purpose only. But this is not to say that Fleming had failed to see the possibility that penicillin might one day be used chemotherapeutically. The eighth of his ten conclusions is quite clear: "It is suggested that it may be an efficient antiseptic for application to, or injection into, areas infected with penicillin-sensitive microbes."

It is strange how Fleming seems to have had this peculiarly ambivalent attitude to his penicillin. It was there, right from the start, because the human conjunctivas which were irrigated every hour for a day and which merely provided evidence for the non-toxicity of penicillin in his original paper were those of Fleming's young assistant, Stuart Craddock. Craddock's importance in the story increases later on, but in the first weeks of penicillin he contributed no more than an infected antrum, which he allowed Fleming to treat by washing out the sinus with penicillin broth. Fleming's laboratory note is quoted by Maurois: "January 9th 1929; mould filtrate antiseptic power on Craddock's antrum. Swab from antrum on blood-agar: 100 staphylococci with myriads of Pfeiffer around. Then 1 c.c. mould filtrate put into right antrum. Swab three hours after on blood-agar. One colony of staphylococci and a few colonies of Pfeiffer. In films as many bacteria seen after as before, but mostly phagocytosed."

The first clinical use of penicillin (though Fleming hadn't even named it then) did no harm and possibly some good, since the antrum infection cleared up. But which was Fleming most interested in: a cure or the persistence of the Pfeiffer bacteria and the disappearance of the staphylococci?

The biography by Maurois also contains one clear memory of a case of "irrigation of large infected surfaces." There was a woman who had slipped and fallen under a bus outside Paddington station. She had a ghastly open wound in the leg, and amputation became necessary. Nevertheless septicemia set in and death seemed inevitable. Fleming, as bacteriologist, was asked his opinion in the normal course of events, and judged the case to be desperate. The source of this information is not given, but apparently Fleming said, "Something very odd has happened in my lab. At this very moment I have got a culture of a mold which destroys staphylococci." He was allowed to try out a dressing soaked in his mold-broth filtrate and applied to the surface of the amputation. But the patient did not recover.

Another of Fleming's assistants, Dr. K.B. Rogers, also provided evidence. An infection of the eye, caused by a variety of pneumococcus, was treated by "mold juice" (as the filtrate was irreverently called). It worked, the infection disappeared, and Fleming was apparently particularly delighted because this meant that Rogers could take part in a shooting match for the hospital team.

Nevertheless, it is clear that Fleming spent less and less time on penicillin after that first paper had appeared. His next published papers in 1929 and 1930 were on other subjects, notably lysozyme. He mentioned penicillin among other things in a paper on antiseptics in 1931, saying simply "It is likely that it or a chemical of a similar nature will be used in the treatment of septic wounds." In 1932 he gave his Presidential Address at the Royal Society of Medicine on "Lysozyme," and since this was an occasion on which he could choose his own topic, it shows clearly where he thought the priorities lay.

A further paper on the use of penicillin in conjunction with potassium tellurite, again with selective isolation of bacteria in the laboratory as the main theme, and a rather despairing paper in 1932 after Harold Raistrick had published his team's failure to isolate penicillin, were his only other contributions in the bibliography of penicillin in these years. This last paper described the treatment of what were called "open indolent septic wounds" with the mold juice; its only words of value today are "It has been used in a number of septic wounds and has certainly appeared to be superior to dressings containing potent chemicals."

Fleming's own story of why he dropped penicillin can be

gained from his own speeches after it had made him famous. In his Harben lectures, given to the Royal Society of Public Health and Hygiene in 1946 he is at his most dour: "We tried it tentatively on a few old sinuses in the hospital and although the reports were favourable there was nothing miraculous. When we asked the surgeons if they had any septic cases they never had any, and then perhaps when they asked us if we had any [penicillin presumably] our whole supply had become inert." He dealt with the matter at greater length in a radio-telephone speech made from London to America when he was replying on behalf of himself and Florey to the presentation of the annual award by the American Pharmaceutical Manufacturers' Association on December 13, 1943:

> However, nothing is more certain than that when in September 1928 I saw on a culture plate bacterial colonies, previously well grown, fading away in the neighbourhood of a mould colony, I had no suspicion that I had got a clue to the most powerful chemotherapeutic substance yet used to defeat bacterial infections in the human body. But the appearance of that culture plate was such that I thought it should not be neglected, so I made pure cultures from the stray mould colony and most of the penicillin hitherto produced has been made from descendants of this one colony. . . .
>
> As I worked with penicillin, however, some of its merits were revealed. It did not affect all microbes—all of the successful chemotherapeutic agents have been selective in their action—it was very diffusible and in the strongest solutions I could get it did not damage human blood corpuscles nor did it cause any poisoning symptoms when injected into animals. To me the absence of toxicity to human leucocytes was very significant, for I had been testing different antiseptics in human blood for years and I had never before come across one which was not more toxic to leucocytes than it was to bacteria.
>
> Here therefore was something to bite on; but when we came to apply the crude penicillin to patients we found we were up against certain snags. The weakness of our unconcentrated solutions gave little or no margin for deterioration, and only on rare occasions did we succeed in preserving the potency of penicillin intact for more than a few weeks.

We tried various simple concentration methods with little success, but as we were mere biologists with no special chemical knowledge this was not surprising. . . . [He then spoke of the work of Raistrick's group which was likewise defeated by the instability of penicillin.] We must recall the conditions prevailing in the early 1930s—little interest was taken in chemotherapy of bacterial infections as everything introduced had been a failure since Ehrlich's Salvarsan and that had been in use for twenty years. Clinicians were getting tired of false alarms. . . .

From 1930 to 1939 I expect that my laboratory at St. Mary's Hospital was the only one where penicillin was in constant use, not for the treatment of patients, but for the isolation of certain microbes—a minor use, but not without value. I still had hopes that someone would purify the active substance and so I did not discard the culture plate on which the original mould spores fell. I have it still, dried up but recognisable.

And that seems to be the nearest Fleming ever came to explaining why he did not follow up the undoubted lead his own acute observation and his very good luck had given him.

Chapter 5
FLEMING— WHAT REALLY HAPPENED

THE TRUTH ABOUT what happened in the little laboratory overlooking Praed Street on that unidentified September morning in 1928 is probably not to be found either in the official biography of Fleming or in his scientific publications. There are other versions of the story.

First there is the myth, so often retold even forty years after the event. As recently as March 25, 1970, a London newspaper carried the headline, bold and simple: "MILLIONS SAVED . . . BY SOME MOULDY JELLY." And the story begins:

> The grimy London dust floated in through a hospital window— and spawned the greatest medical breakthrough of the century.
>
> That breakthrough was penicillin, the first of the antibiotics. Sir Alexander Fleming, who was carrying out research at St. Mary's Hospital, Paddington, in 1928, noticed that some old samples of bacteria which he had cultivated on jelly had gone mouldy

because of the dust. He also noticed that wherever the mould flourished the growth of bacteria had stopped. The mould had killed off the germs. That simple, almost accidental, discovery was the beginning of the era of super, life-saving drugs.

Fleming's first official scientific announcements of his discovery had been greeted with devastating lack of interest by the medical profession. Apart from his scientific publications there was no recorded version of his discovery till after Florey and Chain, at Oxford, had made penicillin a therapeutic drug. But in the later years of the war and immediately afterward there was a spate of newspaper articles and later of books. Probably the most informative of the early works on penicillin was David Masters's book *Miracle Drug*. Published in 1946, nearly twenty years after the moment of discovery, it provides an entirely new witness of the great discovery, a Dr. E.W. Todd, and describes how Fleming had been on holiday in September 1928 and how he returned to his cultures of staphylococci:

> Wishing to find out what sort of growth they had made since he went away he began examining them, glancing at them with an expert eye, casting aside one here and there that had become contaminated by other bacteria which had crept in and were consequently of no further use to him. He was going through those on the window ledge when he picked up one that had a patch of mould about the size of a florin on it. He glanced at it and was about to discard it when something stopped him and made him look at it more closely. His trained eye noted that while colonies of staphylococci flourished all over the medium, around this mould the staphylococci were in the process of being dissolved. He looked again to make sure that he had made no mistake. Then he moved a step or two with the plate in his hand over to Dr. Todd. "Now look at this—this is very interesting," he said. "I like this sort of thing—it might be important."
>
> Dr. Todd looked at the plate. "Yes, very interesting," he agreed and handed the plate back to Dr. Fleming. To tell the truth Dr. Todd was not very impressed. "I thought it was something like lysozyme," he told me.

Next we have the addition of the mold spore coming in through the window. This is well exemplified in *The Life Savers* by Ritchie Calder. The author, now Lord Ritchie Calder, former chairman of the Metrication Board in Britain, was virtually the founding father of my own profession of scientific journalism. He is fairly cautious about the spore, but adds much firsthand observation to the story:

> Fleming's Fluff, which drifted in through a window near Paddington station, belongs, with Archimedes' interrupted bath, Newton's apple and James Watt's kettle-on-the-hob, to the great scientific legends. Those legends have usually a germ (or in Fleming's case a spore) of truth in them, but in the repeated telling they get either over-ornamented or over-simplified. . . . The notion of a micro-organic Tinker Bell skipping in through the window and producing penicillin does less than justice to the shrewd observation and scientific acumen of Alexander Fleming. The setting was certainly unromantic. I knew it well because I used to go there when he was, out of the kindness of his heart, helping me with the bacteriological chapter of a book I was writing. While trains hooted in the adjoining Paddington station and belched their smoke to blacken the laboratory windows and rush hour crowds swarmed noisily below, he would coach me in what I wanted to know. The laboratory was like a museum whose curator had died and the new one had not been appointed. There was labelled confusion. But there were no "museum pieces" in that place; every specimen was working for its living. When the room became stuffy windows had to be opened, and all kinds of living dust invaded the laboratory to ruin the experiments, because the covers of beakers and Petri dishes have to be removed sometimes.
>
> That was what happened in this case. Fleming had prepared a culture of staphylococci for an impending experiment. He had left them to multiply on a nutrient medium and had gone off on a few days' leave. There were many such cultures and on his return he was examining them. The cover of one had shifted and it had been contaminated. To anyone uninitiated it would just have been an experiment which had "gone fusty." There was a growth of mould on it.
>
> Before he threw it away he looked again. He became fas-

cinated because around the mould the germs were not growing; there was a kind of moat. This was the observation of a trained observer, whose sense of curiosity was heightened by the experience of his own previous discovery, made in 1922. This was lysozyme.

Calder, however, is careful to insist that Fleming had not found penicillin in its life-saving form, nor even in any clinically useful form. And later in the same chapter he admits that it was only by a series of coincidences that Fleming's work was taken up again.

But only six years later this story had been transformed by yet another author, L.J. Ludovici. In his *Fleming, Discoverer of Penicillin*, after a whole chapter demonstrating that Fleming had all the qualities needed to qualify as "a great scientist," the mold spore is "directed by the winds of Heaven" to fall on the Petri dish and Fleming is recorded as saying: "A mould spore coming from I don't know where, dropped on the plate. That didn't excite me, I had often seen such contamination before. But what I had never seen before was staphylococci undergoing lysis around the contaminating colony."

Thus, according to Ludovici "a master of his craft with his perceptive genius" spotted that something extraordinary had occurred.

This view of Fleming's significance is difficult to square with the report by Boris Sokoloff in his *Penicillin, A Dramatic Story*, published in 1946. Sokoloff writes: "'When I saw the bacteria fading away,' Fleming said later 'I had no suspicion that I had a clue to the most powerful therapeutic substance yet found to defeat bacterial infections in the human body. But the appearance of that culture plate was such that I thought it should not be neglected.'"

The point I am trying to emphasize here is that Fleming, even according to his own memories, did not *immediately* see the antibacterial, or antibiotic future that might lie in penicillin. He did see this point later and, as his formal publication shows, did suggest back in 1928 that there might be an eventual practical use for penicillin.

It is clear from his scientific papers at the time and from many public speeches in later life that Fleming's own version of his discovery was this: he had spread small numbers of staphylococci over the surface of a standard Petri dish containing a standard nutrient agar mixture and he had incubated the culture in the normal way at 37° C for the usual period of sixteen to twenty-four hours. Under incubation the staphylococci had developed into the usual random scattering of opaque yellowish colonies distributed fairly evenly across the plate. The plate had then been taken out of the incubator and had been left on the laboratory bench for several days or even weeks, being examined at intervals under the microscope. During one of these examinations, which necessitated removing the lid from the plate, airborne mold spores had landed on the surface of the medium and duly developed into colonies of contaminating mold.

One of these colonies had produced penicillin, which had diffused through the agar and attacked the nearest developed yellowish colonies of staphylococci, dissolving (or lysing) them into shapeless, transparent and watery masses. Those colonies of staphylococci further removed from the mold remained unaffected by the penicillin.

The clearest single piece of evidence for thinking Fleming believed this comes from his 1943 speech to the American Pharmaceutical Manufacturers' Association, quoted earlier. The crucial words are these: "I saw on a culture plate bacterial colonies, previously well grown, fading away in the neighbourhood of a mould colony." But there are several supporting quotations from other addresses, such as his Nobel lecture of 1945.

Everyone has assumed that what Fleming saw was a comparatively common event, which other bacteriologists had not recognized as significant or had not been curious enough to follow up. The peculiar luck that had been Fleming's was that the contaminating spore happened to be from one of the very few varieties of penicillium mold that produced penicillin in any large quantity. Florey, for instance, commented: "Quite one of the luckiest accidents that have occurred in medicine, for, without exception, all other mould antibiotics so far examined are poisonous." That was in 1943, when Florey was addressing the Royal Institution, and he said no more about the nature of the finding. Ironically, the work of a scientist who was later to become his wife, was, at that period producing evidence which we can now see carried the implication that Fleming's interpretation of his plate was wrong.

The extraordinary fact is that no scientist could reproduce anything like what Fleming said he had seen on that original plate. For nearly forty years it remained a mystery why Fleming had seen what he had reported seeing. This uncomfortable fact was never revealed by any scientist. And the failure to reproduce the phenomenon seen by Fleming was not for want of trying. Dr. Howard Hughes wrote in 1972 that "our attempts to duplicate the plate for a demonstration have failed until recently."

The man who brought this extraordinary state of affairs to public notice, and who provided a reasonable scientific explanation for what actually happened was Professor Ronald Hare. He had joined the staff of the Inoculation Department just a few months before Fleming made his discovery. Throughout his life Professor Hare has been near to the events of the penicillin story, though never central to them. After some time at St. Mary's he went to Queen Charlotte's Hospital where, by chance, he was closely involved in the early development of the sulpha drugs which prepared the minds of the medical profession for the chemotherapeutic revolution of the antibiotics. He emigrated to Canada and worked at the Connaught Institute, where, by chance again, he became involved in the rather bizarre history of the early development of penicillin on a commercial scale. Finally Hare came back to Britain as professor of bacteriology at St. Thomas's Hospital in London and ended his career as director of a Medical Research Council Laboratory at Carshalton in the southern London suburbs.

It was in his spare time in this final appointment that Hare began to investigate the mystery of the Fleming plate. As the result of his work he showed that Fleming had misinterpreted what he saw on the plate of "mouldy jelly" in 1928. One reason Fleming could not demonstrate his dramatic discovery to inquiring journalists and authors in 1945 and 1946 was that he simply did not understand how to get the same phenomenon to occur again.

Professor Hare began his search for the true origins of penicillin in 1964. He first tried to "rediscover" penicillin in the original way, using Oxford strain staphylococci, which are particularly sensitive to penicillin, and spores from the original Fleming strain of penicillium. He incubated the staphylococci till the fully developed yellowish colonies had been produced and then placed mold spores on the surface with a fine needle at points where there were gaps between the germ colonies. The plate was examined every day and the big surprise was that the mold virtually refused to grow. Normally the mold is not difficult to grow at room temperature if it is seeded onto clean agar plates and it will generally develop a colony some twenty millimeters across in a couple of weeks. But Hare could not get the mold to develop properly on a plate containing staphylococcal colonies. No mold colony would grow to more than ten millimeters across, however long he kept the plate. The vast majority of mold colonies never reached anything like that size, and the only rule that seemed to emerge was that the mold spores seemed to produce better colonies, but still not good ones, if they were planted as far away as possible from any of the well-developed staphylococci.

So Hare went back to Fleming's original paper and studied the picture of the first plate, since no modern prints of the original photograph could be found. Scaling up to the true size of a standard Petri dish he found that the plate showed there were indeed separate, well-developed colonies of staphylococci, each between two to four millimeters in diameter spread over most of the plate in such a way that there would have been about 200 colonies if they had been evenly distributed over the entire plate. But at one edge of the plate was a colony of mold approximately twenty millimeters in diameter, with a smaller colony of mold close beside it. Around the mold was an area about twenty millimeters wide in which there were no developed colonies of staphylococci but sixteen blobs of semitransparent material, the bacteria which had been lysed. Those "ghost colonies" nearest the mold were only from 0.4 to 0.8 millimeters in diameter and those further away were larger, some up to 1.7 millimeters in diameter.

So the next series of experiments was to prepare a large number of plates, each with about 200 colonies of staphylococci on them and try to grow Fleming's mold in the same relative position as it appeared on the original plate. The molds either failed to develop or produced a colony of less than ten millimeters. But by planting the staphylococci in such a way that there was a large empty space in which he could place the mold spores so that there were no staphylococci within ten millimeters, Hare did manage to grow large mold colonies with diameters up to the twenty-millimeter size of the original. But even then *there was no effect on the bacteria,* which continued to look quite normal however long the plate was kept. "No one looking at such a plate could possibly guess that a powerful antibacterial substance was emanating from the mould," writes Professor Hare.

Yet he could easily show with these plates that penicillin was being produced by the large mold colonies and was present in high concentration in the agar. Nevertheless, the staphylococci were undisturbed. The conclusion is plain: "It is extremely improbable that the mould spore can have reached the culture plate [i.e., Fleming's original plate] after the colonies of staphylococci had fully developed, partly because the mould would probably have failed to grow at all and partly because, if it did, the penicillin produced would have had no visible effect on the staphylococcal colonies in its vicinity."

Separate experiments by Dr. W.D. Foster had also shown that penicillin from a growing mold colony does not affect fully developed staphylococci. And Dr. Foster had even tried dropping crystals of pure penicillin onto colonies of the bacteria, so that the concentration of the drug must have been enormous, but they remained unaffected.

In a sense none of this should have been unexpected in

1964 and 1965, for as long ago as 1942 the first evidence had come in that penicillin acts on microbes only while they are young and multiplying; the curative effect of penicillin is achieved by the drug preventing the proper construction of bacterial cell walls, so that the organism literally bursts and spills out all its contents. And again, as long ago as 1944, Lady Florey (then Dr. Margaret Jennings) had shown, in an entirely different type of experiment carried out for quite different purposes, that penicillin from a mold had no effect on fully grown bacterial colonies.

The visible fully developed colony of staphylococci on an incubated culture plate consists mostly of organisms that are already dead or are far beyond that point in their life-cycle where they will multiply and thus be susceptible to penicillin. If there are any young multiplying cells in such a colony they are so few that their death by the action of penicillin cannot be observed by the naked eye. Penicillin acting on young grow- ing cells destroys them completely. But in a half-developed colony of sensitive bacteria penicillin will destroy all the younger cells, leaving the old dead cells unaffected. Such a colony will therefore not disappear entirely, for the dead old cells will still be there to leave some trace of the former exis- tence of the colony and this is, without doubt, the origin of the "degenerate" colonies on Fleming's plate. The colonies that Fleming observed as having undergone lysis were therefore young colonies caught by the penicillin in an early stage of development.

It follows that if the scientist first seeds the mold onto the plate, allows it to grow, and then later seeds staphylococci, he will get a picture like Fleming's, and incidentally this occurs whether or not the plate is incubated. But Fleming in the course of his investigations into the family of staphylococci for his chapter in the nine-volume *System of Bacteriology* would never have tried to culture organisms on a plate already visibly contaminated.

It is possible on the other hand that he was at least trying to grow some staphylococci without incubating them, for it is known that in 1927 he had read a paper by three workers (Bigger, Boland and O'Meara) at Trinity College, Dublin, stating that there were certain varieties of the family which developed in unusual ways, especially as to color if they were grown in unusual circumstances, such as at room temperature.

This gave Hare his next clue. He argued that if the spore of the mold arrived on the plate at more or less the same time as the staphylococci were placed there, or even within a few hours either side of this time, the penicillin effect might be observed if the growth of the bacteria could be postponed. The basic factor here is that the mold grows at much the same speed whatever the temperature (within a fairly wide range of normal), whereas the staphylococci grow very much faster at 37° C (body heat) and hardly grow at all if the temperature is down to 12° C (53° F, which is by no means an unusual temperature in England even inside buildings).

So, on August 1, 1966, Hare performed his crucial experiment. He inoculated a standard culture plate containing nutrient agar with the Oxford staphylococcus, and planted some spores of Fleming's strain of penicillium in one spot on the plate. The plate was put on the laboratory bench, in the shade, but not incubated. By the third day only tiny transparent colonies of staphylococci were visible and they were growing much more slowly than when incubated. But the mold was doing fine; a tiny speck was visible at two days, there was ten millimeters of growth by day four and fifteen millimeters by day six. And in fact on day five it was obvious that penicillin had been "rediscovered" for the first time since the original finding in 1928. "The general picture was indistinguishable from the photograph in Fleming's paper."

On August 15 the experiment was repeated—the correct scientific thing to do—though in an aside Professor Hare declares it was "foolish because it is generally inadvisable to repeat a successful experiment." And this time penicillin was not rediscovered and the experimenter was nonplused. Closer examination showed that both bacterial colonies and mold had grown quite satisfactorily and seemed to be exerting no effect on each other. However, it did appear that the bacterial colonies had matured rather earlier than in the first experiment. The experiment had been most carefully done with full notes taken, and the notes of temperature showed a possible explanation. In the typical manner of an English summer the weather had varied wildly from cold, wet and stormy with an average temperature just above 60° F during the first two weeks of August, the time of the first experiment, to a minor heat wave with temperatures up round 70° F at the time of the repeat experiment. Still it was odd that such a small variance as ten degrees could make all that difference, so a more sophisticated set of experiments was performed.

Three entirely separate sets of culture plates were set up in the same way with mold and bacteria going on at the same time. By now it was the autumn of 1966 and the central heating was switched on in Hare's flat (in Warwick Square, London, close to Victoria station this time). One set of plates went onto the radiators and were kept at 98–99° F. The second set went into the airing cupboard and stayed around 72–74° F while the third set went into an unheated bedroom which was conveniently at 61–63° F. Perhaps amateurish in the way of equipment, but the results were clear enough: penicillin was only "rediscovered" in the bedroom where the temperature was in the 60s. A long series of confirmatory experiments followed. They showed that, although penicillin is almost always "rediscovered" when the temperature is below about 68° F and never shows itself when the temperature is in the 90s, at the intermediate range, in the 70s, many other factors, such as the amount of bacteria originally inoculated and the number of mold spores applied, will affect the result one way or the other. In view of the fact that the original mold was contaminant, and therefore the spores were presumably airborne and few in number, Professor Hare concludes that about 68° F must have been the maximum temperature at which the original process could have taken place. But this would only have been necessary for four or five days at most, because once the mold has grown far enough to start producing penicillin it does not matter how fast the bacteria grow, they will be lysed by the antibiotic.

By now the detective bug must have bitten Professor Hare because he proceeded to call in the help of the Meteorological Office and they provided him with the weather records for July, August, and September 1928. He found that, although there had been a heat wave in mid-August, just as in 1966, it had broken on August 28, 1928, and there had followed nine days of cold weather when the temperature only twice topped 68° F. This appears to fit with the historical uncertainty that no one knows the exact day of Fleming's finding penicillin except that it was probably in the first half of September 1928.

This reconstruction of the likeliest way in which the original penicillin plate came into existence must, of course, always remain a speculation. All that is certain is that it could not have happened in the way Fleming thought it did. If the reconstruction is anywhere near the truth, then Fleming's luck was even more remarkable than is generally believed. For if his discovery did depend on the vagaries of the British climate, then the phenomenon could never have been seen anywhere in the tropics and would have been even more unlikely in countries with the steadier conditions of continental climates, which would rule out the U.S.A., Canada and much of central and eastern Europe.

However, the myth has it that there was extraordinary luck in the fact that it was one particular penicillium out of the thousands of varieties that blew in through the window, and that one was a member of the select few, very few, which produce penicillin in measurable, observable quantities. But when Fleming came, in the course of the experiments reported in his first paper, to test out other varieties of molds to see if they produced penicillin too, he found that all but one failed. That was a strain of penicillium which showed all the characteristics of his contaminant. Where had that similar penicillium come from? Surely not from a second stroke of incredible luck with an open window (a third, if you remember lysozyme).

There is another explanation, quite impossible to prove,

but so reasonable that it seems to demand acceptance. It all started a good many months before Fleming's great moment, when a Dutch scientist, Dr. Storm van Leeuwen, who specialized in allergy, came to London and lectured at St. Thomas's Hospital. One of those who went to hear him (accompanied by Hare) was Dr. John Freeman, that senior member of Wright's department who had first recruited Fleming. Freeman was very impressed by the Dutchman's theory (and his practical results) that molds, common household molds found growing on foundations and floorboards, might cause allergies and particularly asthma. Freeman then persuaded Wright to appoint the Irish mycologist C.J. La Touche (who has already been mentioned in connection with the mis-identification of Fleming's penicillium), with the idea that they could isolate molds from the houses of asthmatic patients, identify and culture them and then inject the patients with extracts from their own household molds in an attempt to desensitize them and thus cure the asthma.

La Touche soon collected a vast assortment of molds, but he had none of the apparatus such as we normally use today, like fume cupboards, in which to deal safely with the enormous number of very light spores produced by the molds. Fleming never mentions the source of his experimental molds, but La Touche has told Hare that the vast majority were given to Fleming by La Touche, and that all of them were identified with La Touche's aid.

Allison has said that he believes that Fleming isolated one mold from a pair of moldy shoes in the studio shed at his country place. Maurois records Fleming asking his fellow members of the Chelsea Arts Club whether they had any moldy shoes or things. But by far the likeliest source for two identical specimens of the same mold in the same laboratory is that they both came from one sample in La Touche's collection.

The circumstantial evidence is strong. The window in Fleming's room would be difficult for so short a man to open, and the window sill was by all accounts usually cluttered with plates and test-tubes. In any case good bacteriologists do not normally work by open windows, for they wish to avoid contaminants. On the other hand, La Touche's room was directly below Fleming's, two floors down, in the same turret, with a staircase and an elevator shaft connecting the two directly. And as the biographers point out, Fleming's door was normally left open. The case against Praed Street and the window is strong.

If La Touche's laboratory was the source from which the mold spore came into Fleming's laboratory, then we can be reasonably sure that the mold in La Touche's laboratory came from the damp basement of some large house in Kensington or Belgravia. It was from such homes of the wealthy that many of Freeman's hay fever patients came and naturally he had collected, or persuaded his patients to collect, the molds from their own homes that might be causing them trouble.

However that may be, the fact remains that Professor Hare's explanation of what occurred in Fleming's laboratory in 1928 is the best modern scientific reconstruction, based largely on technically satisfactory, strictly controlled, modern experimentation. But the first scientific doubts about Fleming's true place and weight in the history of penicillin had been raised, about the time Professor Hare began his piece of detective work, by Professor Gordon T. Stewart, then professor of epidemiology and pathology in the University of North Carolina. Professor Stewart had been working for a time in association with the Beecham Research Laboratories in England where the semi-synthetic penicillins were being developed. In 1965 he wrote a technical book *The Penicillin Group of Drugs*, a book for scientific consumption, unlikely to come into the hands of the public. In the introductory chapter he criticized Fleming for being dilatory in following up his own findings, and he added: "Academic research in medicine is often too fundamental to be concerned with the prevention and cure of disease, but even in sympathetic circles, Fleming's work aroused no interest, nor was there any evidence of exploratory action by the pharmaceutical industry. There are fashions in science no less than in costume; Fleming's observations, reported at a time when therapeutic nihilism was in vogue, were completely ignored."

Professor Stewart suggests that Fleming's inability to communicate and convince might have been a factor in his failure to get encouragement and help in developing his observation of penicillin. The despotism of Sir Almroth Wright could have been a further adverse factor. He concludes: "It must be remembered that biochemistry, wherein lay the solution of Fleming's technical difficulties, was a younger science even than bacteriology. . . . In these circumstances, wittingly or unwittingly, Fleming probably did the best thing he could do in describing, simply and factually, his basic findings; he set the stage admirably for a subsequent performance by a more expert team who read the literature wisely."

In 1968 came Professor Hare's revelations and deductions about the actual nature of Fleming's observations. And then in 1971, to celebrate the thirtieth anniversary of the first clinical use of penicillin, the Royal Society and the Royal College of Physicians organized an international symposium on the latest research on antibiotics and penicillin in particular. The opening lecture was by Professor Chain, now Sir Ernst Boris Chain, professor of biochemistry at the Imperial College of Science and Technology in London. For the first time in public he gave an assessment of Fleming's role, and after referring to the usual "mould through the window" story, he went on: "Fleming indeed had a stroke of good luck, but not in the sense of the commonly presented popular accounts of this event. The phenomenon which Fleming observed seems simple and straightforward enough, but in actual fact it is not, and few people are aware of and understand its complexity and the fact that it needed the coincidence of several most unusual circumstances to make its observation possible."

Professor Chain then summarized Hare's work, obviously approvingly, and went on to emphasize how unusual were the circumstances surrounding Fleming's observation. Modern research has shown that the destruction of staphylococci which

Fleming saw (lysis) was not caused by penicillin, but was a self-destruction (autolysis) of the bacteria which only occurs under very special conditions. He continued:

> The unusual element in Fleming's case was that he left his Petri dish with the staphylococcal colonies on its agar layer for such a long time on the bench that the contaminating mould had time to develop and to exert its antibacterial action on the colonies, and that the colonies were just at the right age and physiological state in which they underwent autolysis under the influence of penicillin. Fleming did not discover the growth-inhibiting effect of penicillin on bacteria *directly* by observing a phenomenon of inhibition of bacterial growth (which penicillin commonly exerts on many bacterial species under many growth conditions and which is, of course, the basis of its chemotherapeutic action) but through a bacteriolytic effect of penicillin which it exerts only under very special conditions, not normally encountered in the bacteriological laboratory and only on a very few bacterial species. Fortunately the staphylococcus on which Fleming had worked was among these. The reason that the antibacterial action of penicillin on bacteria was not discovered long before Fleming, despite its ubiquitous occurrence, was that normally if the bacteriologist sees that one of his plates which he wishes to use for a diagnostic test is contaminated with a mould he does not use it, and thus has no chance of observing an inhibition of bacterial growth by the contaminant; on the other hand once his bacteriological observation is completed, he throws away the Petri dishes as soon as possible without waiting for contaminants to appear.

Finally we have what might be called the official Oxford view of what Fleming did and what was the true importance of his role in the story of penicillin. This is probably the nearest we shall ever come to finding what Florey thought about it, though it was not penned by Florey himself, but was written by Professor E.P. Abraham, who was himself a member of the Oxford team and who still works in the Sir William Dunn School of Pathology at Oxford. He wrote it as part of Florey's obituary in the *Memoir of Lord Florey* of the Royal Society. Noting that Fleming wrote to Florey immediately after the first newspaper reports had appeared concerning penicillin in 1942, Abraham says:

> He [Fleming] added, "You are very lucky in Oxford to be out of range of reporters," but this was not in fact the case. The press sent representatives who received no welcome and little satisfaction from their visit and Florey stated in a letter to Sir Henry Dale that he had taken a firm line. He appears to have had two reasons for this, both commendable in themselves; an inherent dislike of publicity with its distracting effect on research; and the belief that it would lead to a demand for penicillin from members of the public which he could not then satisfy. One result, however, was that the press went where it was not rebuffed and published accounts of penicillin which were tendentious and one-sided, although the facts were mostly on record in the scientific literature.
>
> Fleming, an unusually acute observer, had discovered two substances of major importance—lysozyme and penicillin. In his classical paper on penicillin he had shown that penicillin-containing broth was no more toxic to leucocytes than ordinary broth. He undoubtedly hoped that the substance would be useful for local application to infected surfaces and employed it as a dressing for septic wounds. However, a story later gained currency that he foresaw the importance of penicillin as a systematic chemotherapeutic agent, but was frustrated by the antagonism of Almroth Wright and by the inability of chemists to provide him with a purified preparation for use. This supposed explanation of his inactivity is scarcely credible. No attempt was made to test the chemotherapeutic activity in animals of the concentrates prepared by Ridley and Craddock even after the publication in 1935 of Domagk's experiments with Prontosil, which had shown that a chemical substance could cure otherwise fatal infections by haemolytic streptococci in mice. The attempt of Raistrick, Clutterbuck and Lovell to purify penicillin in 1932 was made at Topley's, not Fleming's suggestion. . . . Fleming at least made no approach to him and stated that he did not know him at the time.
>
> The failure to do animal experiments with crude penicillin may have been connected with the climate of opinion in Almroth Wright's laboratory, for Ronald Hare has stated that these experiments were regarded as artificial and unlikely to produce results which would be applicable to human infections. In any event

Fleming was deterred by the difficulties of isolating penicillin and quickly lost faith in the idea that it might find a place in medicine, since he said in 1940, with reference to its earlier use as a local antiseptic that "the trouble of making it seemed not worthwhile." Five years later he remarked "and now after various ups and downs, we have penicillin." This summary of the work of others in a short and somewhat infelicitous phrase served to strengthen Florey's belief that little attempt was being made to present the story in its true perspective. He had obviously felt tempted on several occasions to make a public statement to this effect, but he accepted the advice of Sir Henry Dale and later of Sir Edward Mellanby (whose letters to him were sometimes fatherly in tone) and did nothing. The advice was sound, for there is no evidence that the judgement of scientific bodies was influenced by popular articles, broadcasts or casual remarks, and all three of those who played leading roles in the story of penicillin received appropriate recognition.

So from the Olympian calm of Oxford, the scurrying writers of the press are rebuffed. If Florey is not given his full meed of praise in the popular mind, and if Fleming is given too much, it is obviously Florey's own reluctance even to "welcome" the press that is to blame. And now the myth seems to have gone too far ever for the truth to be recalled. Shortly after Professor Abraham wrote the obituary there was a play on television in which Fleming was not only depicted as seeing the chemotherapeutic possibilities of penicillin in 1928, but in which Fleming, and not Florey, treated the Oxford policeman, in which Fleming and not Florey soaked his clothes in the mold juice against the day of a German invasion. In a few years Fleming, in myth, may well have taken over all the Oxford work too.

Chapter 6
PENICILLIN
IN ECLIPSE

"It may have been a stroke of good fortune that the spore of *Penicillium notatum* fell on Fleming's plate and attracted his attention by lysing some staphylococci, but the merit of his work lies in the fact that he recognised the changes produced by the fungus, initiated investigation of its properties, and preserved it so that it was later available to others."

This is the summary of Fleming's achievement and place in the history of penicillin written by the Oxford team in 1949, after they had successfully developed the drug from an observation into a life-saving substance. It is in the best traditions of academic objectivity, accurately summing up the true progress made by Fleming and avoiding any mention of those avenues he apparently failed to explore. It is probably a journalistic oversimplification to demand that one man should be named as the discoverer or inventor of each major new development, but certainly this Oxford summary would seem to deny Fleming the right to be called discoverer of penicillin. And that denial is just.

It is true that Fleming injected his mold juice into a healthy animal and showed that penicillin was not toxic to living creatures in very large doses. It is true also that he suggested that penicillin would be useful one day in a chemotherapeutic role. But the question must be asked: Why did he not inject penicillin into a diseased or infected animal? His failure to do so left it to the Oxford team twelve years later. When they carried out this simple experiment the results were so astoundingly successful that it can be claimed that this was the moment penicillin was discovered. For this is what we mean by penicillin: a drug which can be injected into the bloodstream whereupon it will kill invading bacteria by working within the bodily system.

There has never been any answer given to the question: Why did Fleming not try out his mold juice on an infected animal? No one seems ever to have asked him the question. He never seems to have felt any necessity to answer. His own response to the more obvious question as to why there was a twelve-year gap between the first observation of penicillin and its development as a drug was that he had neither the skill nor the staff to tackle the chemical problem involved in purifying and isolating penicillin.

Fleming himself expressed this view many times. In his Nobel lecture he was restrained: "My only merit is that I did not neglect the observation, and that I pursued it as a bacteriologist. The first practical use was to differentiate between different bacteria. We tried to concentrate penicillin but found, as others did later, that it was easily destroyed, and so, to all intents and purposes, we failed. Had I been an active clinician I would doubtless have used it more extensively." Privately he has been reported (by a friend of Florey's) as saying, "I would have produced penicillin in 1929 if I had had the luck to have had a tame refugee chemist at my right hand. I had to stop where I did."

In fact it seems likely that it was in these two omissions, the failure to inject penicillin into a diseased animal and the failure to obtain chemical help, that the general atmosphere of Sir Almroth Wright's scientific philosophy was the real hindrance to immediate progress on penicillin. Experiments on animals were frowned upon as a technique. They were held not to provide results that were relevant to human beings. Chemistry was even less favored.

Wright had declared against having any chemists on the staff long before with a typical dogmatic utterance: "There is not enough of the humanist in chemists to make them suitable colleagues." The structure of the British medical profession and the hospital service of the 1920s was enough to account for the rest. The only serious chemistry that was done at St. Mary's took place in the laboratory of the pathologist, Dr. Roche Lynch, who was mostly occupied with forensic medicine, the search for poisons such as arsenic in corpses and an enormous number of autopsies for the coroners' courts. The only other chemical facilities in the entire hospital were a small basement laboratory where technicians carried out routine blood and urine tests for the clinical staff.

There is no firm evidence that Fleming approached any outside person or body for help with his chemical problems. And it is undoubtedly here that his personal qualities—that lack of persuasiveness, that inability to communicate to which Professor Stewart pointed—held up progress on penicillin. One of those who knew Fleming pointed out: "You have to remember that even if Fleming approached anyone else for help it would have been in a completely offhand way, mumbling almost inaudibly, with the eternal cigarette butt stuck to his lower lip. 'I say, X, I've got something rather interesting in my lab that you might care to look at.' And if there was no response he'd say no more."

But whether he asked anyone or not, it is certain that Fleming did not receive any help from anyone at all outside his own department. Therefore, he summoned what assistance he could from within his own resources. This consisted of two of the young members of the Innoculation Department, Stuart Craddock and Frederick Ridley. Craddock was already Fleming's assistant; Ridley had helped two years previously with the chemical problems of lysozyme, because he, at least, had some chemical training in the shape of a biochemistry course at Birmingham University. But neither man could be called a chemist in the usual sense of the word, and still less had either of them any sort of experience of chemical techniques.

What were the chemical problems that Fleming and his two young helpers faced? Basically they had a broth of meat extracts on which a mold had been growing and which produced some decidedly odd results when it was placed near certain bacteria. They did not know whether there was one active principle which affected the bacteria, or whether there were several different interesting substances in the broth. They had some results showing that the broth stopped bacteria growing near it, and Fleming's original observation (never repeated) that the substance produced by the mold could destroy (apparently) fully grown bacteria. They also had the first evidence that penicillin was unstable; that it lost its power if just stored for a week or two; and that its potency was quite quickly destroyed by fairly moderate heating.

One thing was quite clear: the broth containing penicillin, whatever that might be, could not be directly injected into patients or given intravenously (that is introduced into a vein through a tube) because the broth was a meat broth and therefore contained a large amount of animal protein which would stimulate an intense immune reaction in the patient. Such reaction, which can even cause death from anaphylactic shock, was one of the major problems of the serum-therapy which was so much practiced by Wright, and was, therefore, a clearly understood obstacle to any plans Fleming might have for using penicillin in any way except for washing the outside of wounds or infected surfaces with the broth. It is also at this stage of the development that the meaning of the word penicillin began to change. Originally Fleming had used the newly coined word to stand for the broth with whatever was in it; now the word meant the active substance or substances in the broth.

If one assumes (as we now know to be the case) that the

mold produced one active substance and a variety of other substances, then getting rid of the meaty part of the broth, the protein, would only be one very obvious step toward purification. Getting rid of the water would be another such step.

But real chemical purification, so that one is left only with one substance, and that chemically pure, is a much more complicated business. Nowadays there is a wider set of options open to the chemist approaching a purification problem, but the basic method is to dissolve the complex mixture containing the desired substance in some chemical (it may be distilled water), then to add another liquid (another solvent) which does not react with the first solvent. Some of the chemical substances in the original complex will go into solution in the second solvent rather than in the first. If the two solvents are then separated (perhaps the water may be boiled off) only some fragments of the original complex will be left behind in the remaining second solvent. If the chemist has chosen his solvents well, the different chemical substances in the original complex will choose to go into one solvent or the other according to their chemical nature. Thus all the molecules of any one particular chemical in the original complex will be found in one solvent or the other and not mixed up between both solvents. When the chemist is chasing an unknown substance which shows biological activity, as he might be when trying to purify penicillin, he can find which solvent it has gone into by testing both solvents, after they have been separated, to see in which half the biological activity still resides. In the hunt for penicillin this meant repeating Fleming's type of "ditch" test in an agar-coated Petri dish to see which solvent contained the substances that would stop bacteria growing. Furthermore by comparing the distance from the ditch at which sensitive bacteria stopped growing, with the distance at which they stopped growing when the original broth was placed in the ditch, it was possible to obtain a rough quantitative measure of the amount or strength of the penicillin that had migrated into the solvent.

If the second solvent is found to contain the active principle for which the chemist is searching, he can concentrate the active principle by putting less of the second solvent into the mixture. If, as in the case of penicillin, there was originally very little of the active principle in a large amount of medium, this is a very valuable technique. Another method of testing the strength or concentration of the penicillin separated from the rest of the complex is a reversal of this concentration. By diluting a fixed amount of the residue after separation in increasingly large amounts of water and then using the ditch test it is possible to set up a system of measurement of the amount of concentration and purification that has been achieved.

In many cases, including that of penicillin, a third solvent is then used, added to the second solvent, to split up the original complex even further. If the active principle goes into the third solvent the remains of the original complex can be recovered in a dried form by driving off the third solvent (possibly by boiling again). With any luck the original active principle will be virtually left alone and pure by now. But if there are still contaminants and impurities remaining with it, these will be very similar substances to the one the chemist is seeking. They may only reveal themselves by causing a sudden surge of fever in a patient who has been injected with what the chemist hoped was the pure substance. Impurities of this kind are called pyrogens.

The long struggle to purify penicillin involved all the types of process here mentioned; a good many solvents were tried at various times and the final isolation depended upon a further process of quite a different kind. Because penicillin is so unstable under heating, the final solvent had to be driven off by freeze-drying. Getting rid of a last set of impurities that were, in fact, pyrogens, was one of the later triumphs of Chain and Abraham. But that was still far in the future when Ridley and Craddock started to help Fleming in late 1928.

Both these young men had recently completed their medical studies; neither would have dreamt of calling himself a chemist. Craddock described their state of mind (to Maurois):

> Ridley had sound and pretty advanced ideas about chemistry, but when it came to methods of extraction we were driven back on to books. We read up a description of the classic methods; using

acetone, ether or alcohol as solvent, and evaporating the broth at a fairly low temperature, because we knew that great heat would destroy the substance; working in a vacuum. We knew very little when we began. We knew just a little bit more when we had finished; we learned as we went along.

The detail of what they did was never published until their memories and notebooks were made available to Professor Hare in 1968. This is undoubtedly one of the oddest features of the penicillin story and one of the strangest facets of Fleming's reaction to his discovery. Because Craddock and Ridley did not eventually succeed, it may have seemed not worthwhile publishing their work at the time. But we can now see that they came very near to success and certainly they established a number of major points about the ways of concentrating and extracting penicillin which then had to be rediscovered all over again when later teams tackled the problem. If Chain, for instance, had known the details of their work he might not have set off with an entirely wrong notion of the nature of penicillin; but then if he had not thought the substance was an enzyme, or protein, he might not have been interested in it at all and might never have approached the problem.

The conditions in which the two young men worked were certainly extraordinary. In the biggest laboratory of the department, where they started work, they found that the water pressure in the taps was not sufficient to power the primitive water pump with which they tried to obtain a vacuum. This, they guessed, was because the laboratory was on the second floor. But Ridley then discovered a tap in the corridor near Wright's office, which seemed to be taken directly off the rising water main. This tap flowed into a sink in the corridor where the nurses had washed out bedpans and filled hot-water bottles and kept urine samples in the days when the building had been used as one of the main wards of the hospital, before the Inoculation Department had converted it into laboratories. So it was here in the corridor that they did most of their work. This involved using a very long tube to bring gas out of one of the main laboratories to their work place near the sink. It also involved much squeezing past a disused centrifuge machine which had been parked in the corridor, and which seemed to have a great many angles and projections. The corridor, about twelve feet long and not more than four feet wide, was also very drafty.

Broadly speaking, the work was divided into two main parts; Craddock produced the broth on which the penicillium mold had grown and was also responsible for much of the titration, the tests of the biological activity of the various products of the extraction processes and the measurement of the amount of penicillin contained in the products. Ridley concentrated on the chemical engineering.

The first job was to obtain as much penicillin as possible from the original broth. They used glass bottles or flat-sided flasks lying on their sides, half-filled with broth. They inoculated mold spores onto the surface of the broth and plugged the necks of the flasks with wool. They soon found that if these flasks were incubated at 37° C, body heat, the normal temperature for incubation in bacteriology laboratories, very little penicillin was produced in the broth. So they hunted about the department and found "a large black incubator with a glass door" which they could keep at 20° C, room temperature. They immediately obtained larger quantities of better quality penicillin which would inhibit staphylococci and streptococci at dilutions of 1:600 or even 1:800—that is, one drop of broth in 600 drops of distilled water was enough to stop these bacteria growing in Petri dishes. They also tried to find variations of broth which would produce better growth of the mold or larger production of penicillin. But they found nothing better than "the digest broth of bullock's heart." (Note how their findings about the growth of penicillin at different temperatures might already have provided a clue to the real nature of Fleming's original observation.)

After five days' incubation the broth from the flasks and bottles was filtered through a machine called a Seitz filter. This machine forces liquid through asbestos pads by air pressure which is provided by a bicycle-tire pump working through an ordinary tire valve. It was particularly annoying to use because the reservoir above the asbestos pads held only fifty cubic centimeters of liquid, and so had to be frequently refilled. Nevertheless, it was enough to give them mold juice free from solid particles of the full-grown mold and the bullock's heart.

Then Ridley set about getting rid of the fairly large amount of water in the broth. Because penicillin was so susceptible to destruction by heat he placed the mold juice in a flask, evacuated as much air as he could and heated the flask gently to approximately 40° C. In the partial vacuum the water boiled at this temperature and the steam was drawn off up the vacuum line. The steam also carried away a number of highly volatile substances with it. (At the risk of patronizing some readers: water will boil and turn into steam at a lower temperature than the usual 100° C if the pressure is correspondingly less than atmospheric pressure. This is the reason water boils at lower temperatures high on mountains where the atmosphere is less dense and the pressure less great than at sea level.)

Broadly speaking, Ridley and Craddock were successful at this stage. But to achieve any sort of success they had to make two further discoveries about the process of penicillin extraction which were to remain important right up to our modern mass-production processes. First they found that a great deal of frothing occurred as the broth boiled, and that if the thick frothy bubbles were all drawn away up the vacuum line they lost too much of the valuable liquid along with the steam. Frothing remained an industrial problem even when penicillin production reached the factory stage.

They also discovered the sensitivity of penicillin to the acidity or alkalinity of the medium in which it reposes. They found that their strongest mold juice was highly alkaline, with a pH sometimes as high as 9. (Neutral pH, the measurement of a substance that is neither acid nor alkaline, is 7. A very acid substance has pH 1 and extreme alkalinity is pH 13.)

This alkaline solution rapidly lost all its activity (the penicillin simply disappeared) when the distillation process was tried.

But if they added hydrochloric acid to the mold juice and thus increased its acidity till they reached a pH of 6.5, the penicillin would stay in the liquid and not disappear. They did not know whether the disappearance was due to its departing in the steam or to the actual break-up of the molecules of the active substance. Their discovery of the necessity of acidifying the solution if the active penicillin was to be retained was yet another procedure that had to be rediscovered by others later.

These findings by Ridley and Craddock sound simple enough. In practice they made life almost intolerably difficult. A single distillation took a whole working day; someone had to be on watch all the time to prevent overheating and to see that the water pump attached to the tap continued working and providing a vacuum. Then the discovery that acidification was important led to further problems; the conditions inside the vacuum flask had to be investigated every hour and tested for pH level and further acid added if it was becoming too alkaline. There were no electrical pH measuring devices available in those days; the flask had to be opened every hour and a small sample taken; indicator chemicals had to be added and the resultant color changes had to be compared with charts to measure the pH. They concluded that the entry of oxygen into the flask each time they opened it was destroying the previous penicillin within. Furthermore, after measuring the pH by the clumsy color-change method, they found they often had to add more acid and remeasure the pH, before closing the flask and restarting the vacuum and the heat. So they decided to fill the flask with hydrogen each time they opened it. For this they needed another piece of fairly primitive machinery, a Kipps apparatus, a notoriously temperamental piece of machinery according to those who have had dealings with it.

Taking all this into account it is surprising, and very creditable, that they managed to keep intact most of the penicillin made by the mold in the broth. One of their best days was March 20, 1929. Taking mold juice which gave a strength, a penicillin titer, of 1/100, a sample of 200 cubic centimeters of mold juice was evaporated in the vacuum distillation apparatus to dryness. To the dry remains they added five cubic centimeters of distilled water and the result had a penicillin titer of 1/3000. Considering that the reduction from 200 cubic centimeters to five cubic centimeters is a forty times concentration, this is equivalent to a titre of 1/75 in the original mold juice, so they had lost very little of the original active substance in the process.

Hurdle number one having been crossed, the next step was to remove the proteins and other pyrogens from the dry remainder while trying to keep the active penicillin. The dry remains after the distillation were in fact a brown sticky mess which they described as being like melted toffee.

To this they added acetone, or ether, or alcohol, or chloroform. They soon found that the penicillin dissolved only into acetone or alcohol, and would not go into solution with ether or chloroform. Alcohol turned out to be the most efficient solvent. Ridley's notes describe an experiment on April 10, 1929, only three weeks after the experiment mentioned above. On this occasion 1200 cubic centimeters of mold juice was evaporated to dryness, and dissolved in fifty cubic centimeters of water. To this seventy cubic centimeters of ninety percent alcohol was added and immediately there was a precipitation out of the mixture, i.e., solid particles appeared and gradually fell to the bottom of the flask. This precipitate turned out to be largely the unwanted proteins from the meat broth, and most of the penicillin remained in the mixture of alcohol and water. When the proteins were removed in a simple centrifuge operation the remaining mixture had a penicillin titer of 1/3000, compared with the 1/300 found in the original mold juice.

Vast progress had been made, but a solution of penicillin in almost pure alcohol was quite useless for any serious biological tests, still less for clinical use in medicine. Ridley then drove off the alcohol and water by yet another vacuum distillation treatment. Again he was left with "a small syrupy residue, not more than half a cubic centimeter in volume." This he redissolved in another five cubic centimeters of distilled water and put it in the cranky old refrigerator. Satisfactory, as long as someone remembered to keep renewing the ice.

The titer of activity of this extract was between 1/3000 and 1/5000. So the titer of the little half cubic centimeter of syrup must have been in the region of 1/30,000, which represented real progress.

The work had further shown a number of important facts about penicillin. It seemed that penicillin could not be a protein or enzyme since it had not precipitated out with the other proteins. And since it could remain dissolved in an organic solvent (alcohol) it must be a comparatively small and simple molecule. The extracts kept in the refrigerator retained their activity for only a week or ten days before they started to deteriorate. Therefore, either penicillin was completely unstable or there was still more purification to be done.

So Ridley drove on, with Craddock still helping. He went back to acetone which he had shown was able to take up the original mold juice in solution, though less efficiently than alcohol. He added double the volume of acetone to the samples of syrup left after the alcohol had been distilled off. Again there was a precipitation, and again there was very little penicillin in the precipitate—the penicillin stayed in the acetone. What was in the precipitate was the yellow-brown coloring material that gave the original mold juice and the later syrups their characteristic appearance. This showed that the coloring material was not the penicillin itself but yet another product of the mold. We know now that this coloring matter is chrysogenin, a not very interesting substance. By now they had purified the penicillin even further and concentrated it by a factor of about one hundred compared with the original amount in the mold juice. Ridley's scientific statement of his achievement reads: "By continually adjusting the acidity to pH 6.5 during low-temperature (40° C) vacuum distillation, followed by extraction with alcohol and precipitation of an inactive fraction from the alcoholic solution by two volumes of acetone, this gave us a full yield of high potency penicillin. We lost little in the process."

The next step is quite obvious: to try treating some infected animals with the extracts that Ridley had prepared. There might still be toxic substances left with the penicillin, but they would hardly kill creatures like mice, while the penicillin itself might prove to be active. This is where the weight of the scientific criticism of Fleming must lie.

For nothing was done, Craddock and Ridley were allowed to stop work and not a word about it was ever published except for the statement in Fleming's original paper under the heading "Solubility" where he states: "My colleague, Mr. Ridley, has found that if penicillin is evaporated at a low temperature to a sticky mass, the active principle can be completely extracted by absolute alcohol. It is insoluble in ether or chloroform."

Fleming himself had taken no active part in the work of Ridley and Craddock, but he had quite definitely controlled it and known all about it. Craddock told Professor Hare: "He was 'in' on all we did, but I don't think you can say he directed us in our attempts to concentrate and extract. He tried to help us, but he was as ignorant as we were, and we probably read up the various methods of extracting substances more than he did, and we certainly tried them without his help." He added that Fleming asked for all the titrations that were done and received accounts of them each day on loose-leaf sheets.

It is, then, very odd that Fleming should have said so little about the methods employed when he came to write his original paper. There is no mention of solubility in acetone. There is no mention of the need to employ a vacuum; there is no detail about the temperature employed in the distillation. Still more important is the omission of any mention of the desirability of varying the pH so that the mixture was kept at the acid pH 6.5 all the time. No details were given either, by Fleming, of the titrations at the various stages nor of the possibility of getting a watery solution from the sticky mass produced by the alcohol extraction. And there is no further mention of the work at all in any detail in his later papers or speeches.

The work came to an end in the spring of 1929, barely six

months after the original observation had been made. Craddock, who had just been married, got another job, a better
one, at the Wellcome Research Laboratories in the London
suburb of Beckenham. Fleming did everything he could to
help him achieve this promotion. Ridley likewise wanted to
move as he wished to make himself a career in ophthalmology
(he succeeded in becoming extremely distinguished in his chosen field). But in the spring of 1929 he was suffering from
boils, which none of the vaccines, for which the department
was so famous, could cure. It is an irony that the penicillin
which he was trying to extract would almost certainly have
cured his boils. Instead he went on a cruise to recover, and
then started on ophthalmology.

Fleming seems to have made no attempt to get replace-
ments. It is hard to avoid Professor Hare's conclusion about
Fleming's state of mind, that "by the spring of 1929 he was
losing interest in penicillin as a chemotherapeutic substance
for the treatment of deep-seated infections. It was primarily
for the treatment of this type of infection that the work had
started at all. Why therefore continue with it if the value of
penicillin began to be doubtful?"

Craddock summed up the feeling of depression: "We could
not know at the time we had only one more hurdle to cross.
We had been so often discouraged. We thought we had got the
Thing. We put it into the refrigerator only to find, after a week,
that it had begun to vanish. Had an experienced chemist come
on the scene I think we could have got across that last hurdle.
Then we could have published our results. But the expert did
not materialise."

And so penicillin had to wait another twelve years. And
Fleming, for the while, disappears from the story altogether.

Chapter 7
FURTHER FAILURES

In 1929, THE YEAR that Fleming published his first paper on penicillin, a new department was started at the London School of Hygiene and Tropical Medicine, a Department of Biochemistry. The London School of Hygiene and Tropical Medicine has its buildings in Bloomsbury, just next to the Senate House and administrative buildings of London University, not far from the back of the British Museum. Its original motivation came, of course, from the existence of the British Empire in so many parts of the tropical world, and even nowadays it continues to do much work for, and with, the less developed nations. Much of its research work has also been concerned with those diseases and disease organisms which are mostly found in tropical countries. But it has never been strictly bound to operate within the subjects implied in its title; industrial diseases and hospital administration are among the many subjects in which it specializes at the present time.

The new Department of Biochemistry naturally had to have a distinguished biochemist at its head, and Professor Harold Raistrick was chosen. He stipulated, however, that he should be allowed to carry on his work with molds, and this was accepted. A solid Yorkshireman, Raistrick had by 1929 already specialized in the study of molds and had discovered sixteen chemicals previously unknown to science which were produced by various different molds in the course of their growth. He was to become one of the greatest mold-chemists in the world of science and by the end of his career he had discovered more than a hundred new chemical substances, all of which came from molds.

This background is significant because the attempts by Raistrick and his team to isolate penicillin are invariably presented as a direct and logical follow-up of Fleming's original discovery, a second assault on the mysteries of the mold, another determined attempt to give the world its first antibiotic. This is hindsight, and it does not correspond to the objectives of the researchers at the time the work was done.

Raistrick's department was only founded in the year that Fleming published his original observations. It was two years later that Raistrick looked into the penicillin mystery and then he did it as part of his own systematic research into the world of the molds and as part of his lifework of examining the chemicals produced by molds. When penicillin proved elusive, Raistrick simply abandoned the problem and made no attempt to carry out the crucial biological experiment of trying out fairly well-concentrated penicillin on animals infected with bacteria that penicillin was known to affect.

But when he decided to look at "The formation from glucose by members of the *Penicillium chrysogenum* series of a pigment, an alkali soluble protein, and penicillin—the antibacterial substance of Fleming" (this is the title of the scientific paper recording the investigation, which was published in 1932 in the *Biochemical Journal*), Raistrick collected a strong team. He had his own assistant, Dr. P.W. Clutterbuck, a biochemist; he borrowed the services of Dr. Reginald Lovell (who later became a professor in his own right), a bacteriologist from Professor W.W.C. Topley's Department of Bacteriology directly upstairs from him; and he had a mycologist, Mr. J.H.V. Charles, working on the same problems.

Fleming was asked to provide specimens of his penicillin-producing strain of penicillium from St. Mary's. Fleming obliged most willingly, but his only other contact with the work was a number of telephone calls to Dr. Lovell. There is no trace of Fleming ever having asked Raistrick to do this work, and it seems that the two men did not even know each other at this time. Certainly Fleming told them nothing about the work done by Craddock and Ridley, and Professor Hare supplies the almost incredible piece of information that Lovell, the bacteriologist of the team, knew nothing about Ridley's work at all until Professor Hare told him about it, thirty-seven years after it was completed.

So Raistrick and his team started virtually from scratch. Raistrick himself did very little of the work and left most of it to Clutterbuck, Lovell, and the mycologist, Charles. They first confirmed Fleming's original work; this is not an example of distrust but a proper scientific procedure. They then obtained further samples of Fleming's strain of penicillium from the Lister Institute, as well as examples of a similar mold *Penicillium chrysogenum* which had originally been discovered by the American mycologist, Dr. Charles Thom. From Dr. Thom himself they got examples of *Penicillium notatum* which had first been discovered on moldy hyssop in Norway by Westling. In their turn they sent specimens of Fleming's mold to Dr. Thom.

Fleming's mold, it must be remembered, had been identified as a *Penicillium rubrum*. But Charles Thom decided it was in fact a variant form of *Penicillium notatum;* that is to say, it looked like *Penicillium notatum* but in its reaction to different growth media it differed from the standard form. It was able to grow happily on milk; if grown on gelatin it precipitated a brilliant yellow coloring material like the *Penicillium chrysogenum;* it grew particularly well on a diet of glucose. But Raistrick's team showed that neither *Penicillium chrysogenum* nor the original form of *Penicillium notatum* from the Norwegian hyssop produced penicillin, or at least anything that could be found to stop the growth of germs.

The correct identification of Fleming's penicillin-producing strain of penicillium as a variant of *Penicillium notatum* was one major step forward. Raistrick's next contribution was undoubtedly his most important. He showed that Fleming's penicillium could be grown on an artificial medium. The original bullock's heart broth was both expensive and difficult to prepare, furthermore it was naturally subject to slight variations in content which made later measurements of activity and penicillin production difficult to calibrate.

It took a couple of months' work by Raistrick's team to show that Fleming's mold would grow on a standard laboratory medium, known as Czapek-Dox medium (named for the two scientists who invented it). This medium simply consisted of distilled water with a fairly straightforward admixture of cheap mineral salts. Modified by the addition of glucose—the mold's favorite food—the Czapek-Dox medium proved quite satisfactory, for although the mold grew more slowly on it than on the meat broth, it eventually produced higher concentrations of penicillin.

Clutterbuck was mainly responsible for the first reasonably large production of penicillin in the laboratory. He put the modified Czapek-Dox medium in a hundred flasks and steamed the flasks three times over three days to ensure sterility before injecting penicillium spores. He ended up with some eight gallons of dark brown liquid on which a major program for extracting penicillin could begin. Here we must remember that Raistrick and his team were much more highly qualified and skilled chemists than Fleming and his assistants. Clutterbuck quickly spotted the point about alkali and acid. The dark brown liquid was slightly alkaline; so, very slowly, he added sulphuric acid in small quantities, and immediately a yellow pigment collected in flakes, precipitated and was easily filtered off. This was, of course, chrysogenin, and not penicillin, as was quickly proved by Lovell who showed that the yellow material had no action against bacteria while the antibacterial activity remained in the fluid that had been filtered off.

The credit for the discovery of chrysogenin goes to Raistrick and his team, for they published their results for the rest of the scientific world. The fact that chrysogenin had been found by Ridley and Craddock at a different stage of the purification process remained unknown until Professor Hare unearthed it, and published it forty years later.

That Raistrick was not leading a great assault on the mystery of penicillin with a view to presenting the world with a new drug is quite clearly shown by the record at this point. Far from discarding the inactive chrysogenin and concentrating on the active fraction containing penicillin, they concentrated their work on the coloring material.

First they found that if they added the sulphuric acid to the original brew of mold juice quickly instead of slowly, there was no precipitation of yellowish flakes, and they could not isolate the chrysogenin at all. Then they found that their yellowish material was soluble in ether, but they could not make it crystallize. They used more sophisticated solvents, ending up with ether-nitrobenzene-diazomethane mixtures. They were eventually able to separate out a reddish-brown impurity and to characterize dihydrochrysogenin as $C_{18}H_{24}O_6$; they were even able to make preliminary suggestions about its structure.

Next they extracted a protein from the penicillin-containing brew. This is the alkali-soluble protein mentioned in the title of their eventual paper. (The proteins that Ridley and Craddock had to remove came from the bullock heart, and were not, therefore, present in the mold juice produced on the artificial Czapek-Dox medium.) This protein, too, was analyzed and characterized by a similar steady, but lengthy, process. Only after the protein had been dealt with did Raistrick return to the penicillin.

This long delay had one good result. They learned quite a lot about keeping penicillin in a fairly active condition in the juice while they struggled with the other products of the penicillium mold. At the peak of its production of penicillin the mold was giving a titer of 1/1280, that is one drop of mold juice in 1280 drops of water would stop germs growing. This production peak occurred on the sixteenth day of growth on the artificial medium (it had been between five and eight days on Fleming's broth). The test organism in the Raistrick work was no longer Fleming's staphylococcus, but was the pneumococcus germ, which Lovell, the bacteriologist of the party, chose because he was familiar with its workings.

Mold juice of this strength, stored in an ice chest at zero degrees, would lose half its strength in seven days, and then seemed to stay at about the same level for a further three weeks. By the end of the third month of storage the titer was down to 1/320, only a quarter of its original potency. Even this loss was fairly encouraging by the standards of those days, but what was really disturbing was the ease with which the stored juice became infected by airborne bacteria and totally ruined. It was in an attempt to defeat this contamination problem that Raistrick's team found out how to store penicillin juice. Once again they added a little acid to bring the slightly alkaline original juice to a state of slight acidity. Stored in ice at this acidity the juice kept its full potency for three months at least, though any samples taken for testing purposes had to be brought back to neutrality by the addition of alkali before any biological tests could be done.

Faced, eventually, by the task of concentrating and purifying the juice to find the antibacterial substance, the Raistrick team had to rediscover what Ridley and Craddock had already found out: to evaporate the water even under vacuum conditions they had to have the mixture slightly acidic, pH about 6. But as opposed to Craddock and Ridley, Clutterbuck had already made his juice much more acid than that in the process of getting the chrysogenin out, so he had to add some alkali before he could evaporate the water away. And then he found a bonus. At this acidity the remainder of the extract was soluble in ether. Fleming, of course, had reported that penicillin was not soluble in ether, but this was because he had been using the original alkaline mold juice. Once again it is the crucial question of the pH of the medium that decides which way the penicillin will move.

The great advantage of having the penicillin in an ether solution should have been that ether is very easy to get rid of, as it simply evaporates away in ordinary dry air. This is just what the Raistrick team tried; they blew a blast of dry sterilized air over the solution of penicillin in ether. The ether vanished —but the penicillin disappeared too!

This was a quite unprecedented happening. It astounded these experienced biochemists. Raistrick said, "Such a thing was never known to a chemist before. It was unbelievable. We could do nothing in the face of it, so we dropped it and went on with our other investigations and experiments." So ended the second assault on penicillin, an assault which was never intended as such. Raistrick was interested in molds, not in antibiotics.

A little was rescued from the ether catastrophe: they found that if they added water to the ether-penicillin solution and then evaporated the ether, some of the penicillin was left behind with the water. But the strength was only a quarter of the original and it did not seem worth pursuing.

Raistrick can hardly be accused of having failed with penicillin, because he did not set out to do what the others, before and after him, attempted, which was to find a chemotherapeutic substance. But when nine or ten years later he saw what he had only just missed he developed, according to those who knew him, a curiously ambivalent, and entirely understandable, attitude. He would vary between bitterness over his lost opportunity and self-justification on the grounds that it "was not his job." And when he was asked, apparently point-blank by David Masters, why he had not pursued his experiments he "was averse to discussing the matter."

Lovell, however, was engagingly frank when Masters asked him the same question in 1945. He was then deputy director of the Research Institute in Animal Pathology of the Royal Veterinary College. "I remember making a note in my card

index to try penicillin on mice infected with pneumococcus,"
was Lovell's remark, and he promptly went to the card index
and turned up two references to other men's work on pneumococcus which were marked in his handwriting. "(N.B. for penicillin filtrate)"—in other words, reminders to himself to try the
crude penicillin concentrate on infected mice.

But these are might-have-beens. What happened when the
penicillin proved so elusive, when Raistrick was turning back
to his own firmly held line of work, was that his team of assistants broke up, in part tragically.

The first blow was the tragedy of the young mycologist, Dr.
J.H.V. Charles, being run over and killed by a bus. This distressing incident occurred at precisely the time when Clutterbuck and Lovell were correcting the proofs for their major
paper on their work, the 1932 *Biochemical Journal* report. Then,
in the latter half of 1932, Lovell was appointed to the staff of
the Royal Veterinary College. In professional terms this was
a promotion, but in penicillin terms it deprived the team of its
bacteriologist.

In later years Fleming gave a fairly constant explanation of
the "failure to produce penicillin." In his chapter in the *History
and Development of Penicillin* there is a good example. "I had
failed to advance further for the want of adequate chemical
help. Raistrick and his associates had lacked bacteriological
cooperation, so the problems of the effective concentration of
penicillin remained unsolved." We have seen that the first
sentence is barely adequate recognition of how near Ridley
and Craddock came to success. The second sentence cannot
be upheld at all. Professor Hare, for instance, is quite blunt.
"It is very doubtful whether any of this is true," he writes.
Certainly Raistrick had a fully qualified bacteriologist on his
team, and in fact Lovell did not physically leave to take up his
post at the Royal Veterinary College until the autumn of 1933.
And just as Fleming could have found chemists if he had really
tried, so could Raistrick have found other bacteriologists. It is
worth repeating therefore that Raistrick did not "fail" to isolate and purify penicillin as it seems to us now, he simply did

not set out to try to do this because this was not his interest.

The truth of the matter is that there was no long struggle to unmask the mysteries of the mold because no one in the early 1930s conceived the possibility of an antibiotic as we know it now.

To keep the record straight, it must be added that when a young chemist named Lewis Holt joined the staff of the Inoculation Department at St. Mary's in 1934, Fleming did ask him to have another "shot" at purifying penicillin. It was not given first priority by Fleming, and he did not even mention Craddock and Ridley's work to his new assistant, though he did advise him to read the paper by Clutterbuck, Lovell and Raistrick. For a few weeks Holt tried, using amyl acetate as the solvent because it would not mix with water. This is interesting because amyl acetate was used in the final solution to the problem, but Holt, like the others, was baffled by the instability of penicillin and gave up without publishing anything. Fleming did not press him to persevere.

Only one man in the whole of America appears even to have noticed Fleming's original paper. He was Dr. Roger R. Reid, of the Division of Bacteriology at the State College of Pennsylvania. He started work on penicillin problems in 1930, which must have been very shortly after Fleming's paper became available in the U.S.A. Reid tackled the situation very thoroughly, very scientifically. It seems to have been sheer bad luck that all the answers he came up with, although time has shown them to be correct on the whole, were negative answers.

He started by studying as many varieties of mold as he could, to find if any other produced a substance like Fleming's. Again Dr. Charles Thom was called in, to provide mold specimens, including Fleming's strain, and to identify others. But after examining twenty-three different types of mold, Dr. Reid could find nothing like penicillin among their products. Then he set out to find if the nature of the medium on which the mold was grown affected the action of penicillin against germs, using his own variation of the ditch test. The results were inconsistent and confusing, which no one nowadays would consider surprising with our greater knowledge of the variability of penicillin. Reid also studied the germs that were affected by penicillin and those that were insensitive to it, trying to find any common factor in either of the groups. He could find no common factor.

But in a development of this work he showed that penicillin did not lyse, or destroy, bacteria as Fleming said he had originally observed it doing. Reid found that on laboratory plates penicillin would only stop germs growing. It was, technically, only bacteriostatic and not bacteriolytic or bactericidal. This was a foretaste of the discoveries Professor Hare was to make thirty years later, but it hardly amounted to a matter of controversy in the 1930s when penicillin was such an obscure subject.

Reid then showed that penicillin was inactivated by ultraviolet light, and an attempt to speed its growth by bubbling oxygen through the medium ended with the opposite of the desired result: no penicillin at all.

Finally, although Raistrick's 1932 paper was well known to him, the American elected to have a shot at isolating the penicillin himself. He used methods different from Raistrick's, relying mostly on filtering through collodion bags. He isolated chrysogenin in this way, and for a short while was led up a blind alley here. But he was eventually forced back to the use of acetone and ether solvents, and he got no further than any of the others; indeed he did not get as far, for he never managed to achieve solubility in ether at all. Reid was still working at penicillin in 1935, but then the attention of everyone who was interested in chemotherapy and drugs was attracted by a totally new arrival in the field, a "breakthrough" if ever there was such a thing.

The first human medical cases to be cured by penicillin were three babies and a colliery manager. The cures were recorded in 1931, a year in which Fleming still had some hope and interest left in penicillin; the year in which Raistrick and his team were working flat out on the products of the penicillium mold; the year after Reid had just started work in America.

Yet these cases were never published in any medical journal. They remained quite unknown and unrecognized until penicillin became famous, when they were discovered by investigating journalists and authors. In fact, it was almost certainly David Masters who brought them to light.

The work was done by a young doctor, Dr. C.G. Paine, who was at that time doing hospital bacteriology in Sheffield, the Yorkshire city which is the steel capital of Britain. Paine had been a pupil of Fleming's at St. Mary's during his medical training. He was not asked by Fleming to do the trials of penicillin, but he spotted the original paper on penicillin and was interested by it. He wrote to Fleming and simply asked for some specimens of the mold, which Fleming, as always, willingly supplied.

Entirely on his own, Paine started off by repeating Fleming's work and finding that the mold did, indeed, produce an antibacterial substance in the broth. He used as his test germ a staphylococcus that he had isolated himself from a carbuncle. He even worked out a primitive unit of measurement, based on the distance from the mold juice at which the growth of the staphylococcus was stopped.

When he had collected enough mold juice Paine tried it out on his first three experimental patients. They were all cases of persistent staphylococcal infections of the skin, referred to him by the dermatologist. It seemed to Paine (as it had seemed to Fleming independently at St. Mary's) that this sort of surface infection which could be treated by applying dressings of the antibacterial mold juice was the ideal way of proving the value of penicillin. We know now that they were wrong, and that antibiotics, as a general rule, are best used systemically: taken into the bloodstream through the mouth or by injection so that they can attack the invader throughout the whole living system. But the meat broth which Fleming and Paine possessed was, in any case, quite unsuitable for injection.

Certainly Paine's first three cases were not successes by any measurement. After seven days the treatment with dressing soaked in mold juice was discontinued with the patients showing no improvement. Fleming had had similar results and could only say that the penicillin did no harm. Paine looking back on the three cases said, "The results were uniformly disappointing." In view of the low penicillin content, and the presence of nutrient material in the filtrates, it is not surprising that no good results were obtained.

But with different types of infection Paine's results were much more promising. At the same time as the skin cases were failing to respond even though fresh dressings were applied every four hours, four Sheffield babies with eye infections were providing the first known examples of penicillin's curative power. Two of the four babies were infected with staphylococcus and two with gonococcus, the germ of the venereal disease gonorrhea which they had contracted from their mothers during birth. The mold juice filtrate was applied to the babies' eyes once every four hours. And within three days three of the babies were cured.

The response of the gonococcal infections was particularly remarkable. It was not until the mid-1940s that penicillin was officially hailed as the cure for gonorrhea, following the work of Dr. Wallace Herrell at the Mayo Clinic in the U.S.A., and a large-scale trial in the U.S. Marine Hospital on Staten Island when all but four of 129 patients were completely cured. The gonococcus was one of the original germs which Fleming had shown to be sensitive to penicillin and the American work provided a major proof of the value of penicillin. This makes Dr. Paine's results even more remarkable, and their failure to make any impact at the time even more sad.

Of the two babies with staphylococcal infection, one was cured within three days. The other did not respond to the treatment at all. No explanation could be offered at the time for this difference and one is left wondering whether the uncured baby had the first recorded example of a strain of staphylococcus that was naturally resistant to penicillin. The problem of natural resistance of bacteria to penicillin and other antibiotics was later (in the 1950s and 1960s) to become a major cause of concern. If it was first exhibited in this Sheffield case, then Sheffield did indeed exhibit a fascinating and prophetic microcosm of what was to come. But it went unnoticed and unregarded.

Dr. Paine had one further, and even more impressive, case. This was the colliery manager, whose eye had been penetrated by a small chip of rock when he was down the mine. The wound then became infected and when he was brought to the ophthalmic surgeon it seemed as if he might lose the sight of the eye. The eyeball and eyelids were so swollen and infected that it seemed that the usual delicate operation for removal of the offending stone sliver must be impossible. Swabs from the infected areas of the eye showed a pure culture of pneumococcus which, of course, is normally associated with causing pneumonia, but which is also known to be capable of severely damaging the eye if it can gain access to the interior of the eyeball.

But pneumococcus was also one of the bacteria known to be sensitive to penicillin from Fleming's first experiments. So it was decided to let Dr. Paine try his mold filtrate. Forty-eight hours of continuous irrigation of the eye with the mold juice completely wiped out the pneumococcus. The operation for the removal of the stone chip went ahead normally and successfully and the colliery manager's sight was saved.

And that was the last time that Dr. Paine used penicillin. The basic reason for his disenchantment with the substance was the difficulty he was having manufacturing the mold juice in any regular way. Some brews would show a strength of nine units in his crude method of calculation; but the next brew, for no discernible reason, would have a strength of only two units. The molds also showed quite uncontrollable variations and mutations. One line would produce good quantities of penicillin for a couple of generations and then, all of a sudden, refuse to produce any more. This problem of random mutations in the productive strains of *Penicillium notatum* continued to be a cause of concern, and much irritation, well into the years of industrial production.

So Dr. Paine's own summing-up of his story reads: "The variability of the strain of Penicillium and my transfer to a different line of work led me to neglect further investigation of the possibilities of penicillin, an omission which, as you may well imagine, I have often regretted since."

But the fact that the first humans were cured by penicillin in Sheffield in 1931 and nobody took any notice, is not the only paradox in this short section of the history of penicillin. There is an even more extraordinary coincidence to be found in Sheffield in 1931. The professor of pathology at Sheffield University in that year was a young Australian, Dr. Howard Florey, soon to move on to the post of professor of pathology at Oxford University. Not only were Dr. Paine's experiments done right under Florey's nose, so to speak, but Florey was actually told by Dr. Paine of the results he had achieved, particularly against the gonococcus.

Florey, however, insisted that this clue which was offered to him in Sheffield did not lead to his later decision to investigate penicillin in Oxford. He seems to have forgotten it completely until his own success with penicillin in 1941 reminded him of the discussion ten years previously. And it is the proof of Florey's honesty and self-awareness that it was he who told Masters in 1945 to look up Dr. Paine, the forgotten man who had first cured a human by using penicillin.

Chapter 8
THE CONCEPT OF CHEMOTHERAPY

To THOSE OF US who live in the 1970s there are two aspects of the early part of the penicillin story that must seem very strange: that Fleming's fellow scientists were so unimpressed by his observations, and that the pharmaceutical industry showed no desire to develop his findings. At least four major scientific papers dealing with penicillin appeared between 1928 and 1935: two from Fleming himself, one from Raistrick and his colleagues, and one in America from Reid. All these papers made it clear that they were dealing with a substance that killed bacteria, yet no other scientists and no drug company followed up the lead.

The reason the scientists did not follow up what may seem to us an exciting discovery was that they lived and worked in an atmosphere that was wholly opposed to the very concept of chemotherapy. A substance which could kill bacteria in the test-tube or laboratory dish was thought unlikely to kill bacteria in the body without killing the body cells at the same time.

The reason the pharmaceutical industry did not follow up the observations of penicillin is even more clear. The pharmaceutical industry, as we know it today, did not exist in the late 1920s. It was penicillin and the other antibiotics which brought the modern drug industry into existence. Every modern drug company has its own laboratories in which information scientists scan all the literature, and in which huge numbers of compounds are monitored by automatic programs to see if, by any chance, they exhibit biological activity which could be put to use or profit. But this has only come about because penicillin was discovered and developed through the chance observation of its biological activity.

Of course, there were some drugs and medical chemicals being manufactured on a large scale in the early 1920s, aspirin and phenacetin being the two most obvious examples. And there were Ehrlich's arsenic-based cures for syphilis, Salvarsan and Neo-Salvarsan as the only known synthetically made specific cures for a disease, the first true chemotherapeutic agents. The discovery and preparation of insulin by Banting and Best in Canada also dates from the early 1920s. Yet most insulin and most of the vaccines in use in that decade were prepared by research institutes rather than by pharmaceutical companies, just as the Inoculation Department of St. Mary's Hospital manufactured vaccines.

A few figures will establish the point. In the mid 1930s the total sales of the entire drug industry of the U.S.A. amounted to some $250 million. Twenty years later, in 1959, the American drug industry sold $2 billion worth of ethical drugs (those not advertised to the public) and $450 million worth of proprietary drugs (those which are publicly advertised).

The U.S. Pharmacopoeia, that is the list of drugs and medicaments available to the medical profession, contained on average only six new substances or preparations each year from 1905 to 1935. In the next ten years to 1945, the average number of new drugs added each year was 37. In 1955 the new edition contained 73 new drugs added in that single year.

The situation in Britain in the 1920s was little short of desperate. The 1914 British Pharmacopoeia listed just 80 synthetic drugs, mostly of the aspirin and phenacetin families, and all but a few were imports from Germany. *A History of the Modern British Chemical Industry,* by D.W.F. Hardie and J. Davidson Pratt, states that the basic cause of this situation was the failure of Britain to develop a strong and diversified dyestuffs industry. The Germans developed such an industry (largely based on the inventions of the British chemist, Perkins), and the knowledge of organic chemistry thus obtained provided the basis for the rise and development of the German synthetic pharmaceutical industry from the 1880s onward.

In 1924 the entire output of the British drugs and pharmaceutical industry was worth £15.2 million, and by 1937 it was still only worth £21 million. By 1948, despite the intervention of World War II, the pharmaceutical industry in the U.K. was selling £73 million worth of drugs each year.

But in the period of the first observation of penicillin the entire chemical industry of the U.K. seemed to be on the verge of collapse. In 1920 the government had to take urgent steps and it passed the Dyestuffs (Import Regulations) Bill. In the words of Hardie and Pratt this was "to prevent the threatened destruction of the U.K. dyestuffs industry."

And these were precisely the years when the entire chemical industry in Britain was reorganized and strengthened by voluntary mergers. I.C.I. Limited, the largest chemical company in Britain, and one of the largest in the world, was formed by merger in 1926 and began active operations in its new form only in 1929. So the company which might be regarded as most likely to have provided finance and support for the development of penicillin was only in process of formation when penicillin was first observed. At this same time other British companies which were later to be deeply involved in penicillin production were barely recognizable as what we should now call pharmaceutical companies. Glaxo, for instance, was mostly involved in the baby-food and medicated-food fields. The main interest of the Distillers Company is obvious in its name. The one hopeful factor was the interest that these and similar companies were showing in the manufacture of synthetic vitamins, following the work of Sir Ernest Gowland Hopkins at Cambridge, which showed the necessity of vitamins in trace quantities for proper nutrition.

In fact the only great organic chemistry industry anywhere in the world in the 1920s was on the banks of the river Rhine. The Swiss chemical companies were centered around Basle and some of them are today among the largest pharmaceutical companies in the world. Further down the Rhine valley were the German companies such as Bayer, Hoechst and I.G. Farben Industrie. They had behind them the knowledge of Ehrlich's painstaking search for his effective arsenical compounds, and, despite years of disappointment, there were still chemists and bacteriologists in Germany who believed that continuing the search would provide more "magic bullets." The "magic bullet" was Ehrlich's objective: a chemical which would attach itself to specific bacteria and destroy them, just as dyes and stains would attach themselves to specific bacteria and reveal them under the microscope. It was only in the Rhineland that one could find, in the 1920s, research programs deliberately seeking new biologically active substances.

The U.S. pharmaceutical industry was, however, beginning to look like the modern idea of a drug industry by the mid 1930s. A really large-scale effort to deal with pneumonia, so often a fatal condition forty years ago, was being mounted, based on the claim that if the right vaccine were administered within thirty-six hours of the disease starting, a patient was fairly sure to recover. Vaccines against the thirty-two different types of organism known to cause pneumonia, many of them varieties of pneumococcus, had been produced in the laboratory. All over the country special diagnostic centers had been set up for the identification of specimens from pneumonia patients, more than 2500 centers in all. Instructions had been issued to traffic police to speed such specimens through from the doctors to the diagnostic centers. Five of the country's major drug firms were occupied with the research and preparation for mass production of the vaccines. Lederle had built themselves the world's largest rabbit-breeding station in the course of the work. But nevertheless the situation remained thus: "A pneumonia patient given a reasonable environment and nursing care, probably stood almost as good a chance of recovery in the days of Galen as he did in 1935." The words were written by Dr. Wyndham Davies, M.P., in 1967 as the opening sentence of his book *The Pharmaceutical Industry.*

The breakthrough that opened the way to chemotherapy and made all this American expenditure on vaccines irrelevant came in 1935 in Germany. Breakthrough, but not by penicillin.

The great American plan to defeat pneumonia by vaccine therapy, the plan that was never finally to be fulfilled, would have been the greatest demonstration of the approach to medicine advocated by Sir Almroth Wright. But its collapse proved to be the final defeat of Wright's doctrine: "The doctor of the future will be a vaccinator."

The pneumonia vaccine plan was killed by the arrival of the first of the sulphonamides, the sulpha drugs, which were the first general purpose chemotherapeutic agents. There were, of course, plenty more vaccines still to come. The polio vaccines are probably the most famous of the later ones. But in broad terms what has developed is that we still rely on vaccines to protect us against virus infections, against which we have virtually no drugs, while we have come to rely almost entirely on drugs to deal with bacterial infections. And the breakthrough into this chemotherapy came with the sulpha drugs.

Breakthrough is a word so grossly overused that it has become a joke. But to describe the coming of the sulfa drugs it is justified. The greatest effect of the sulpha drugs lay, not so much in saving lives that previously could not have been saved, but more in breaking the mold of standard thinking in the medical world. By their obvious effectiveness in many cases and against many different organisms the sulpha drugs opened medical minds to the possibility of chemotherapy. The sulpha drugs also proved the value of drug research to minds outside the medical world. They achieved the revolution in thought which was necessary to allow the antibiotics to be developed.

The first sulpha drug was announced to the world by Dr. Gerhard Domagk, director of research of the German Bayer company which was itself a subsidiary of the giant I.G. Farben Industrie. The announcement came in the form of a paper in the *Deutsche Medizinische Wochenschrift* of February 15, 1935, entitled "Ein Beitrag zur Chemotherapie der bacteriellen Infektionen." The drug was called Prontosil and it was in simple fact a dyestuff which had been developed by the company's vast array of research chemists, a rich red-golden coloring material which had turned out to have remarkable curative properties when examined by Domagk, the bacteriologist. He discovered that Prontosil would not kill bacteria in a test-tube, but it would cure living mice that had been given lethal infective doses of hemolytic streptococci.

The development of the sulphonamides is relevant to the story of penicillin more for their effect on the minds of men than for their effect on the bodies of patients. The revelation of the existence of the first sulpha drugs was rather unsatisfactory and has led to the asking of questions which are still unanswered. Why was Domagk's discovery only published in 1935 when the work was done in 1932? Why had 1500 patients been treated in Germany with sulphonamides before the announcement was made? Was I.G. Farben Industrie deliberately delaying the announcement of their find in the hopes of being able to discover a patentable product?

Domagk's methods were simple enough, though heroically thorough by the standards of the times, with no automation and no computer to help. He rejected the current doctrine that it was more economical to try the action of new chemicals against bacteria in the test-tube alone. It had been noted in his own laboratory that some substances were active against bacteria in the living bodies of animals even when they showed no activity against bacteria in the test-tube. No one knew why this should be so, and none of these substances proved clinically useful. But Domagk determined to miss no chance, and so everything was tested in live animals. He thus reverted to the methods by which Ehrlich had discovered Salvarsan, though Ehrlich had no alternative to using live animals since he could not culture his spirochetes, the organisms causing syphilis, in test-tubes on artificial media. These substances that acted in the body rather than in test-tubes were named by Domagk and his colleagues as "true chemotherapeutic substances" to distinguish them from the antiseptics which simply destroyed bacteria and body cells without discrimination.

Incidentally, Sir Almroth Wright visited Domagk's enormous research establishment at Elberfeld in the Ruhr near Düsseldorf and was positively shocked by what he saw. Wright described his visit over the famous library tea-table at St. Mary's and Professor Hare remembers: "Blind groping in the dark in this way was so utterly foreign to someone of Wright's temperament that he looked on it as a form of sacrilege. To him the only method was to think the thing out in the privacy of one's study and then do the experiment to prove the theory." Which throws a little further light on Fleming's attitude and his omission of the biological tests when he could not purify the active substance.

Domagk had tested many compounds based on metals such as gold, tin and antimony, and of course he had tried arsenic compounds. But any that showed activity against bacteria were always too toxic to be of any clinical promise. Then he turned his attention to the azo-dyes that his company chemists were producing. Prontosil was the result of an attempt to get a new dye that penetrated more deeply into the fabric and was therefore more color-fast against the effects of light and so on. It was but one of the azo-dyes developed with this object.

When Prontosil was injected into the stomach cavities of mice one and a half hours after they had been given an injection in the same area with hemolytic streptococci, twelve treated mice survived for seven days whereas all fourteen untreated control mice died within four days. This was the essence of Domagk's discovery, the nub of his first paper. He also published simultaneously two papers describing clinical use of the new substance.

Within nine months of the publication of Domagk's report the problem of why Prontosil acted against bacteria in the body but not in the test-tube was solved by the French husband-and-wife team, Dr. Jacques and Madame Trefouel. They showed that the chemicals in the living body broke down the Prontosil molecule into two different components, and that it was one of these components, sulphanilamide, which attacked bacteria when it was liberated from the rest of the dye molecule. Their work was confirmed by Dr. Albert Fuller in 1936 when he showed that sulphanilamide was being excreted by the kidneys of patients being treated with Prontosil. Sulphanilamide had, in fact, been discovered many years before, in Vienna in 1908 by Paul Gelmo, then working for his doctoral thesis. No one in those days had thought of testing it as a drug, but its discovery prior to 1935 meant that it could not be patented as a drug.

There are nearly as many ironies in the sulphanilamide story as there are in penicillin. Hindsight shows that as early as 1919, two Americans had claimed that certain azo-derivatives of sulphanilamide (i.e., substances exactly of the type of Prontosil) had shown antibacterial action in the test-tube. But the action was so weak that they had not pursued it. Gelmo had passed on from his doctorate at the Vienna Institute of Technology to become an analytical chemist for a firm of printing-ink manufacturers after World War I. Domagk's first human patient was his own daughter Hildegarde, who had pricked her finger with a knitting needle and developed septicemia. She thus posed her father an agonizing problem, but he showed faith in his own work and she was cured by the sulpha drug.

Because sulphanilamide was a simple chemical long known to science there was no possibility of the German company patenting their findings and making a financial killing out of the new drug. This in turn meant that chemists in the research departments of other companies could be easily turned onto the sulphonamides in attempts to produce better, more active versions of the original substance. This turned out to be of particular importance in Britain, where pharmaceutical research was lagging seriously behind the efforts of the Germans and the Americans because of the basic weakness of the organic chemical industry.

But before this spurt in research could come about, the sulpha drugs had to exert their vital effect on the thinking of the medical profession. It is surprising how small a body of men had to be influenced before the whole weight of medical opinion started to swing in favor of chemotherapy. Many of the people involved in the dramatic change of thought that occurred in 1935 and 1936 were those we have already met in the course of the story of penicillin: Colebrook, Fleming, Topley, Hare.

We have seen that Sir Almroth Wright had already visited Domagk at work, and not liked what he saw. Fleming, however, quickly switched to the new subject and his published papers of the period 1937 to 1940 are all on the subject of sulphonamides.

Outside Germany the man who did most of the early convincing work on sulphonamides was Leonard Colebrook, who was working at St. Mary's in Wright's department at the time of the observation of penicillin. Since then he had moved to Queen Charlotte's Maternity Hospital in West London where he led a team doing research into puerperal fever. The immediate connection with Prontosil was that puerperal fever is caused by the hemolytic streptococci, the very organisms against which Prontosil had first proved its value. Ronald Hare was one of Colebrook's chief assistants at Queen Charlotte's. It seems almost incredible that so few men should have been so closely involved with the same story. Time and again, by what seems mere chance, their lives and the story of penicillin cross and recross. The explanation is not chance or the influence of the stars, but the less dramatic fact that at any one time there are probably not more than two or three hundred men dominating any one branch of science. The members of this peer group communicate with each other unofficially and very rapidly and therefore are usually among the first to follow up each other's new moves.

Professor Hare describes the news of the sulpha drugs

coming to Britain in the shape of a post card to Colebrook from his friend Dr. Claud Lillingston, who worked in Paris and regularly kept them in touch with developments in Europe. Lillingston's post card did little more than give a reference to Domagk's paper, and Hare decided to leave it until Colebrook returned from his summer holiday. Hare's reaction, in fact, was "Another of those damned compounds from Germany with a trade name and of unknown composition that are no use anyway." He goes on to explain: "What I thought on this occasion may bring home to those who did not live through this period what bacteriologists thought about chemical compounds for the treatment of bacterial infection. None of us, not even the inhabitants of the Inoculation Department, were, as Maurois supposed, hostile to them. But we were, time and again, infuriated by the claims put forward by clinicians and commercial firms for compounds that should never have been introduced into medicine at all." Some of the disappointments most freshly in his mind at that time were mercurochrome, Sanocrysin and antivirus.

Colebrook did, however, go further and looked up Domagk's paper in the library of the Royal Society of Medicine, and found one or two other not very impressive German reports on the same subject which had appeared by then. Then in October 1935 Professor Heinrich Hoerlein, director of the Bayer Laboratories and one of the chemists who had originally produced Prontosil as a dyestuff, came to London to lecture at the Royal Society of Medicine. He was able to give some more details about Prontosil and the work done on it in the medical field. It was only after his visit that Colebrook was able to obtain some small quantities of the drug, which the Germans seemed very reluctant to part with. In the proper scientific manner Colebrook set about confirming Domagk's work by repeating the experiments, and he soon found, too, that Prontosil had no effect in the test-tube.

"He therefore had to do what everyone in the school of Wright hated doing, test the compound in mice. Not because of any dislike of vivisection, but because the current doctrine was that infection of animals by injecting organisms was so artificial a proceeding that any lessons learned as a result would probably not be applicable to naturally acquired human infections. The causation and pathology of such infections were judged to be very different."

And at first sight it seemed as if Wright's doctrines were justified. Colebrook took six different strains of hemolytic streptococci, all of which had been isolated from human mothers suffering from puerperal fever, which was often a fatal condition. And Prontosil showed no effect against the streptococci in mice. Prontosil was very nearly dropped there and then.

But at the crucial moment there was a visitor to Queen Charlotte's from the Wellcome Research Institute, Dr. G.A.H. Buttle who likewise was working on Prontosil. He told Colebrook that more virulent strains of hemolytic streptococci had shown susceptibility to the drug in his laboratories at Beckenham. He supplied Colebrook with the more vigorous strain of bacteria and Colebrook was able to satisfy himself that Prontosil worked, at least in some cases. Thereafter the conviction that Prontosil was going to be really useful was supported by most of Colebrook's intense program of tests, and by Christmas 1935 Colebrook himself was beginning to feel that he was on to something good.

Three weeks later Ronald Hare had the dubious pleasure of being one of the first human beings outside Germany to be treated with Prontosil. In the course of his research into puerperal fever as part of Colebrook's team, Hare had pricked his finger with a sliver of glass that was contaminated with streptococci. Within a couple of days it seemed unlikely that he would survive and he was in St. Mary's Hospital again, but this time as a patient. Colebrook himself administered Prontosil intravenously and by tablet. Hare turned bright pink as the dyestuff went into his system and "felt so much worse that I began to wonder whether I was dying because of the drug or the microbes."

Fleming, always the best and truest of personal friends,

visited the bedside, and appeared to share the patient's self-diagnosis because when he met Hare's wife he simply, laconically remarked, "Hae ye said your prayers?" Hare recovered in about ten days and, what was even more unusual, recovered the full use of the infected hand. It was while he was convalescing, or losing his bright pink color as he prefers to describe it, that Colebrook really started using Prontosil on mothers suffering from puerperal fever.

Colebrook was faced with a difficult decision. To obtain statistical proof of the efficiency of Prontosil in human cases of infection with hemolytic streptococci the ideal way is to treat only half of the sample cases with the drug and leave the other half untreated so that the true activity of the drug is not masked by chance variations among other factors. In the case of puerperal fever this was, scientifically speaking, even more desirable because the disease can be caused by the several different variants of hemolytic streptococci, *Streptococcus pyogenes*, with different degrees of virulence and severity. Milder, but sometimes still fatal, cases can also be caused by other organisms.

But could one apply the strict scientific protocol to distressing infections which killed sometimes more than two out of every thousand women who had babies and made many more seriously ill, sometimes with crippling after-effects? The death rate in cases infected by some of the worst types of streptococci was more than twenty-five percent.

Colebrook took the humane decision, though this left the controversy to run more lengthily in the end. Basing himself on his own and his team's ability to give remarkably accurate prognoses of the likely course of the disease when they observed the clinical condition of patients as they were brought in, he began to treat those patients who seemed most to need it with Prontosil. This was, as Hare says, "depending more on art than science," but Colebrook had more experience of puerperal disease than probably anyone else in the country. And Hare remembers the growing excitement: "I was no more than a spectator, but I soon sensed that a change had come.

Patients whom we would have given up before, now recovered easily and without the long drawn-out desperate illness that would have previously been their lot. In consequence there were only three deaths among the thirty-eight cases treated in the first six months of 1936, and none at all amongst another twenty-six admitted during the second half of that year. A death rate of only 4.6 percent for streptococcal infections of the puerperium was unheard of." Colebrook himself used the words: "Something we had never seen before in ten years' experience of the disease."

Colebrook with his chief clinical assistant, Maeve Kenny, published the most exciting of their results in the *Lancet* on June 6, 1936. And this, if anything, simply broadened the controversy over Prontosil. The same issue of the *Lancet* carried an editorial urging the greatest caution in accepting the results. Professor W. Topley, Raistrick's colleague at the London School of Hygiene and Tropical Medicine, who had loaned Raistrick the services of Dr. Lovell for his investigation of penicillin four years before, was openly suspicious of Prontosil. In particular he criticized the lack of satisfactory statistics. Topley, described by Hare as "the bacteriological pontiff of the country at that time" adopted such an attitude that "If he had had his way, it is improbable that anything further would have been heard of it."

The chief argument used by the anti-Prontosil school was that for some unexplained reason the hemolytic streptococci were suddenly losing their virulence in the natural course of events. (This argument is by no means ridiculous: there is very good evidence that the organisms causing most cases of diphtheria and scarlet fever in our own time are naturally less virulent than those that circulated in our communities before World War II.) The evidence on which this view was based was that in the first half of 1936 the death rate from puerperal fever at the North-Western Fever Hospital in Hampstead, a suburb of London only five miles away from Queen Charlotte's, had been only 5.26 percent, extraordinarily low for those years. Supporters of Colebrook produced evidence that the women admitted to Hampstead had been less seriously infected than those brought to the specialist hospital of Queen Charlotte's.

The controversy was at its height when the Second International Congress of Microbiology met in London in July 1936, just a month after Colebrook had published his first results. The news about Prontosil and the revolution in thinking can really be said to have started at this congress. To the congress came Dr. and Mme. Trefouel, from the Pasteur Institute in Paris, with their work which demonstrated how a dye could also be a drug and how the active principle was really sulphanilamide. Just before the congress opened, Dr. Albert Fuller had done his work of confirmation by finding sulphanilamide in the patients' urine. The patients in question were those mothers at Queen Charlotte's whom Colebrook was treating, for Fuller was the biochemist in Colebrook's team.

The main day for discussion of the hemolytic streptococci was July 28, 1936. At this session Dr. Perrin Long, of the Johns Hopkins Hospital in the U.S.A., described his work on producing antisera to the streptococci. The aim was to produce vaccines against such infections in the tradition of Almroth Wright's work, although it could even then be foreseen that such vaccines produced in rabbits would be fantastically expensive. The last speaker of the morning was Colebrook. He was supposed to talk about anerobic streptococci, but at the last moment he changed his mind and described his results with Prontosil. The audience was impressed by his sincerity but quite manifestly not convinced that they were in at the start of a revolution.

During the afternoon Hare teased Perrin Long by asking him what he was going to do with his expensive antisera now that Prontosil was doing the job. Long plainly had no idea what Hare was talking about, and it turned out he had not even heard Colebrook's talk. Instead he had been visiting the other American expert on hemolytic streptococci, Dr. Howard Brown, also from Baltimore, who had suddenly found himself a patient in a London hospital because he had forgotten that in Britain there is a left-hand driving rule. The results of the meeting between Hare and Long were dramatic and fully confirmed the traditional picture of American "hustle." Long immediately canceled his proposed trip on the Continent and cabled to the pharmacy department of Johns Hopkins to obtain Prontosil and sulphanilamide by any means whatever. He then took the next boat home, having introduced Hare to the delights of bourbon whiskey while obtaining an account of his personal experience with Prontosil. On arrival in the U.S.A. Long found no Prontosil available anywhere, but at least the DuPont Company was preparing a special delivery of what was apparently the only sulphanilamide outside Europe. By the first issue of the *Journal of the American Medical Association* of 1937, Long was able to report the cure of infected mice with sulphanilamide and the first human cures in America: a case of erysipelas in a child, a case of puerperal fever and several other less severe complaints such as quinsy and ear infections.

Further progress with sulphanilamide was less spectacular, but steadier. It was established that it was effective against some germs but not against others. It was likewise shown that it was effective, not by killing bacteria directly, but by interfering with the life cycle by a process involving stealing the enzymes which the bacteria needed for development. This in itself was an eye-opener to the scientific world of the day, which had not been able easily to visualize how a chemical could render bacteria harmless without killing body cells in the wholesale and indiscriminate manner of the antiseptics.

Chemists in many research laboratories turned their attention to sulphanilamide. Their approach was identical to that of the dyestuff chemists. They took the basic molecular structure of sulphanilamide and by processes of trial and error added different side-chains (i.e., other small molecules or structures of atoms which could be persuaded to attach themselves to the sulphanilamide molecule). Then they tested the resultant substances to find if they were more powerful as drugs than the original. Many new sulpha drugs were produced this way, and a few possessed notable advantages over sulphanilamide and were taken up by the medical profession. The most successful was produced by Dr. A.J. Ewins, a gentle-mannered research chemist working for the British firm of May and Baker.

May and Baker was then, and still is, a comparatively small firm by the standards of the international pharmaceutical giants. It has a strong connection with the agricultural world, particularly with the horticulturalists and market-garden industries just to the east of London where the firm itself is based. It was one of the first British pharmaceutical companies to build up a small research team, and Dr. Ewins himself had been in touch with Colebrook shortly after World War I when St. Mary's had been carrying out an unsuccessful campaign to see if the arsenical compounds would provide anything useful other than Salvarsan.

It took Dr. Ewins three years' work and the testing of no less than 692 derivatives of sulphonamide, before he found success with his 693d variation of the theme. So the new drug was called M&B 693, more popularly just M&B.

Technically this was sulphapyridine, that is to say a pyridine, a six-membered ring of carbon, hydrogen and nitrogen atoms attached to the much smaller sulphanilamide molecule. It was particularly effective against the pneumococcus germs, and it earned world fame in a very short time as the drug which twice saved the life of Winston Churchill during the war years. Despite the success of M&B 693 the May and Baker team went on to synthesize a further 3000 compounds on the same lines but found that only five or six showed any useful activity. Other firms produced other variants and the production of new sulphonamides (to give them their family name) still continues.

Nor was the lesson missed by companies which had no research teams. It cannot be without significance that I.C.I. set up their first pharmaceutical research department in precisely the year 1936. There were just eight scientists in the first group.

The stimulation of pharmaceutical research was undoubtedly one of the important effects of the coming of the sulfa drugs. But their effect on thinking was much broader than this. Professor Hare emphasizes just how important it seemed to one of the men who lived through the breakthrough:

> The fact remains that his [Domagk's] was one of the most important medical discoveries that has ever been made, for it not only enables us to treat and cure a whole series of very serious forms of infection, but of even greater importance, it showed us how wrong had been our ideas about how a successful chemotherapeutic agent was likely to act. As a consequence of this, penicillin began to be thought of as a possible alternative. But let there be no doubt about it, without the sulphonamides to show the way, it is improbable that penicillin would have emerged from its obscurity.

Chapter 9
ANTAGONISM

IN 1939 PENICILLIN was no more than one of a large class of observations of a phenomenon known as bacterial antagonism. This means no more than the fact that the presence of one micro-organism can inhibit or prevent the growth of another micro-organism. There is competition among different species in the world of bacteria, microbes and molds just as there is competition for food supplies and living space among the macro-organisms of animals, birds and plants. Many micro-organisms produce chemicals which inhibit or destroy their competitors.

There had been several attempts to harness the phenomenon of bacterial antagonism to medical use in the eighty years between Pasteur's first demonstration of the existence of germs and the start of World War II. All had failed. Early French bacteriologists had even used the word antibiosis to describe the phenomenon of antagonism between micro-organisms, since the word means "working against life." The word fell into disuse and was only revived in 1941 by Dr. Selman A. Waksman, the discoverer of streptomycin in the U.S.A., who coined our modern word antibiotic. By a strange chance the word which means "working against life" has therefore become the description of drugs which work most strongly against death, at least as far as human beings are concerned.

The first established report of bacterial antagonism as a scientific observation came from Joseph Lister, the surgeon, in 1871. This was followed in 1877 by one from Pasteur. Working with Joubert he showed that anthrax germs did not flourish and grow in animals and cultures where some much commoner and less virulent germs were present first. In a sense there was nothing surprising in this. There was no reason to suspect the newly discovered micro-organisms of not competing with each other just as the larger visible insects and animals and plants competed with each other. And Darwin had not only explained this competition but, in a sense, had justified it.

Pasteur was one of the leaders in the hunt for bacteria that would destroy other types of bacteria. But as more success was attained by his methods of immunization, he left the field eventually and tended to favor the idea that immunization and bacterial antagonism worked by depriving the infectious germs or the less successful of the bacterial antagonists of some essential food substances (rather than by the two quite different mechanisms which we now accept, immunization working by stimulating the body's own immune mechanisms and bacterial antagonism working by the production of an antibiotic).

The first major successes came in the 1880s in Germany. It was found possible to protect rabbits against anthrax by giving them an injection containing a bacterium of the streptococcus family. Then another bacterium named *Micrococcus anthratoxicus* was found which produced a substance that prevented the growth of anthrax germs. Neither of these lines of research was developed much further because Pasteur had developed a highly successful method of immunizing animals against anthrax by using a vaccine containing dead anthrax germs, and had proved his point in a famous public experiment at Melun in 1881.

Yet another clue was provided by experiments with a different kind of micro-organism, *Bacillus pyocyaneus*. It was found that if animals were injected with this germ at the same time as they received anthrax organisms, they would suffer only a slight fever and recover quickly. It seemed that *Bacillus pyocyaneus* protected the animals in some unknown way. In 1898 two Austrian scientists tried to apply this finding to human use. They grew large quantities of the bacillus in culture fluids and then filtered the result very carefully to extract all the living bacteria, for they believed it was a substance produced by *Bacillus pyocyaneus* rather than the organism itself which killed the anthrax germs. This was the first attempt to use an antibiotic on humans. With the filtered fluid they started to treat patients suffering from ulcers on the legs by soaking bandages in the fluid and keeping the ulcers saturated with it. They soon had favorable results to report on over a hundred cases of patients treated with this fluid, including some whose ulcers had been so bad that it had seemed that the limbs must be amputated. They went on to even larger scale trials of the fluid.

A year later, two German scientists announced that they had obtained from *Bacillus pyocyaneus* a substance which they named pyocyanase and which they claimed had the power of dissolving not only anthrax germs but diphtheria germs as well. The two sets of results were quite independent, so there was considerable excitement about this promising new product. Pyocyanase became much used for the treatment of all sorts of external symptoms of infection from boils to gonorrhea. The vogue for pyocyanase lasted for at least ten years, until well into the present century. Doctors continuously reported good results from it, but then for some reason began to drop it. When the commercially available product was tested scientifically in 1929 it was shown to be completely inactive against all germs. The likeliest explanation of the decrease in popularity of pyocyanase (and this popularity was almost always confined to the Continent) and its eventual total inactivity, is that the original strain of bacillus underwent one or several mutations which resulted in its producing less active substances than the originally discovered pyocyanase. This judgment is based on hindsight because the variability of the penicillin-producing strains of the penicillium molds and their liability to sudden mutations which stopped them producing penicillin was one of the great problems in the early days of penicillin investigation. There is another important parallel to be drawn here with the early days of penicillin, in that all the applications of pyocyanase were external, applied to boils and inflammations and ulcers and the like. This was exactly the way in which Fleming started and the results were most disappointing. The concept of applying a remedy systemically (that is, inserting it into the body so that it will attack the invading germs throughout the whole system) had not yet dawned on any of the users of pyocyanase. Nevertheless, the evidence in favor of pyocyanase as a scientifically significant example of bacterial antagonism was every bit as strong as the evidence for penicillin.

In the early years of the present century it was also discovered that molds, too, could produce antibiotics or at least antibacterial substances. In 1913 the mold *Aspergillus fumigatus* was tested and it was found that a culture fluid in which this mold had been grown would destroy the tubercle bacillus in the test-tube. Injections of the fluid were given to patients suffering from tuberculosis, but without successful results. Modern biochemical research, using techniques far beyond anything available in 1913, has shown that *Aspergillus fumigatus* produces at least four antibacterial substances, fumigatin, spinulosin, gliotoxin and helvolic acid.

The molds were a subject of much interest to scientists in the first decade of this century and the years immediately before; this was the time when the molds were first really thoroughly examined. In 1905 the Royal Society in London, the foremost British scientific organization, had invited Professor Ward Marshall to give a review lecture on the molds in which he summarized the then state of knowledge of this family of creatures and mentioned some of the most exciting work going on in the field. His lecture contained one very specific reference to the penicillia. He pointed out that the injection of spores of penicillia and other molds into the brains of kittens produced very rapid death. Apparently the distinguished Professor had not noticed or had been unimpressed by some Italian research that now seems to be the most important early work on penicillium molds and their products.

It seems quite possible that the first recorded scientific observation of penicillin in action may have been made, not by Alexander Fleming, but by an Italian, Dr. B. Gosio, in 1896. He was investigating cases of pellagra among the workers of the agricultural areas of northern Italy. This is a disease which we now believe to be caused by faulty diet, but Gosio suspected it might be caused by infected corn. In a long series of studies he examined many of the rusts and molds that can be found attacking the ears of corn (incidentally, this is to use the word corn in the American sense, or what the English call maize). He found no fewer than fifteen different organisms infecting the corn of which the most important he considered to be *Penicillium glaucum*. Gosio cultured his *Penicillium glaucum* on all sorts of different liquids, including some which are very similar to the media used forty years later for cultivating our modern strains of penicillin-producing penicillium molds. He found in due course that the culture medium would stop the growth of anthrax germs in the test-tube. He got similar results when he cultured another variety of penicillium which we call *Penicillium brevi-compactum* (because it has very short sporing organs).

Of course, Gosio had neither the equipment nor technique to take this work much further. Perhaps more important, he did not have the funds either, and in any case this was not the objective of his research. He thought the penicillium molds were causing the pellagra cases, and the only antibacterial substance he could find in his cultures of penicillia was mycophenolic acid. Today this is known to be an antibacterial. But since it is also known that many different forms of penicillium mold produce penicillin, even if only in very small quantities, and since there is some doubt about the exact identification of the molds with which Gosio was working, there is an outside possibility that he had, in fact, seen penicillin in action.

Fifteen years later (1913) at the same time as the first results were obtained with the aspergillus mold, two British scientists took up Gosio's work and produced more of the mycophenolic acid from the penicillium molds. They even injected it into mice and showed that it did no harm. Working with a closely related mould, *Penicillium puberulum*, they produced a substance which they called penicillic acid. This turned out to kill the *Bacillus coli* which is an extremely common inhabitant of the human intestine, but when injected into mice it proved fatally toxic, and it was therefore never tried on human beings.

Another fifteen years was to pass before the next significant entry about penicillium molds would be found in the literature of medical research. The author of the paper in 1928 was, of course, Dr. Alexander Fleming. And he was quite adamant that none of this previous work had been in his mind when it came his turn to observe the antibacterial action of a culture fluid in which a penicillium mold had been grown. In 1945 he acknowledged the existence of much work on bacterial antagonism before him, but declared "None of the older work had any influence on the birth of penicillin."

When penicillin became a household word, Dr. André Gratia, professor of bacteriology at the University of Liège in Belgium, remembered that in the early 1920s, probably in 1924, he had seen the action of *Penicillium notatum* on a culture plate containing staphylococci. Gratia had been working with his associate, Dr. Sara Dath, at an annex of the Pasteur Institute in Brussels, engaged on a vast survey of fungi and molds. The conditions under which the mold spores contaminated the plate of bacteria were very similar to those in Fleming's case, and the incubation must also have been similar. Even the area of inhibition around the growing mold looked very like Fleming's. But Gratia and Dath, with their primary interest centered on another line of research, made no more than a brief note of the phenomenon.

Gratia often spoke of his missed chance and held himself up to his students in his lectures as a prime example of a man who failed to pursue an unusual biological phenomenon to its full understanding. Fleming's claim to glory is that he did something about what he saw; he preserved and cultured the mold, he investigated its activity and he published his results for other scientists' knowledge and profit.

One final example of bacterial antagonism deserves mention. In Australia, working for the New South Wales Linnaean Society at Sydney, a bacteriologist named Grieg Smith noted in the mid-1930s that a class of soil organisms (called actinomycetes) exhibited antibacterial activity in the classic tradition of bacterial antagonism. His publication started the trail of research in the U.S.A. which led through the discovery of actinomycin to the development of streptomycin by Waksman. This line of work proceeded parallel to and quite independent of the penicillin development and is, in itself, a fascinating example of the fact that many important scientific developments have often occurred in two different places, simultaneously and quite independently.

In Oxford the research program that was to lead to the development and the giving to the world of penicillin as a drug —the first of the antibiotics—began as a piece of pure scientific research, an investigation of bacterial antagonism as a natural phenomenon. The men who began that program were Howard Florey, newly appointed professor of pathology at the Sir William Dunn School of Pathology of the University of Oxford, and Dr. Ernst Boris Chain, his newly recruited biochemical expert.

Chapter 10
THE TRIUMPH
OF PENICILLIN

AT OXFORD Florey and Chain did not set out to produce penicillin. Like any other good scientists in a university department they wanted to carry out a program of first-rate scientific work. They wanted to produce new and interesting results, relevant to the general body of medical and biochemical knowledge of their time.

But they were short of money; they could not afford the technical assistance, the instruments and the equipment that they needed to press on with their work. This is a situation well known to almost all scientists before and since. So they set out to create a program of research for the department that would be attractive and successful in gaining sponsorship and support from fund-providing organizations outside and beyond the usual sources on which Oxford men were wont to call.

Work on the antibacterial substance that had been noted as produced by the mold *Penicillium notatum* was but one item in a proposed study of the whole field of bacterial antagonism.

Work on several other apparently similar substances was just as much in their minds. The study of bacterial antagonisms was only half of their original program and equal priority was given to the other half. They chose to include penicillin in their list because they believed it to be something quite different from what it turned out to be. They considered that penicillin was an enzyme, a protein, and as such it lay directly in the field they had already been studying. Had they known that it was a small and simple molecule they would not have considered studying it. They set out to study it not because it might turn out to be a useful drug; even at quite a late stage in the process their primary aim was to find out the mechanism by which it produced its curious effect. This was simply a logical development of their earlier purely scientific work on other substances.

Yet eventually the scientists of the Sir William Dunn School of Pathology of Oxford University made four quite crucial achievements which together amounted to giving the world the first antibiotic: penicillin. Their four achievements:

1. To show that penicillin was a usable clinical drug with powers of curing infection that were beyond the wildest dreams of man no more than forty years ago.

2. To isolate and purify penicillin to a state in which it could safely be used for human patients. (It was only several years later that they succeeded in producing completely pure penicillin crystals.)

3. They carried out the first clinical testing of penicillin on humans, and in so doing saved many lives in the course of their scientific program.

4. They found out how to manufacture penicillin on a commercial scale. They manufactured considerable quantities of the drug themselves, and provided know-how to both British and American pharmaceutical companies for all the early production of penicillin that was used by the fighting men of both Britain and the U.S.A. (The superiority of the deep-fermentation method of producing penicillin—which was the unique American contribution to the story of penicillin—only became clear in about 1945.)

The first two of these achievements were the proper work of a university department. The third might be considered marginal. The fourth achievement was a quite extraordinary departure from the normal activities of research workers in a university by the standards of those times. It was still more extraordinary by the standards of Oxford University which remains to this day a somewhat conservative fortress of "pure" academic standards. The least-recognized part of the achievement of Florey and Chain and their fellow workers was their adaptability, their willingness to forsake their chosen fields and their normal roles when they were faced with the fact that they had something quite unprecedented in human experience on their hands: nothing less than the most powerful drug that man had ever found.

It was in this aspect of the Oxford work that Florey particularly earned his claim to greatness. He had not only led his collaborators through the scientific stages of the inquiry; he was also the man who flew off to America to get the help that could not be provided in wartime Britain; he was the man who threw himself into the world of government committees and supply priorities to start production going at home; he was the man who went out to the battlefields of North Africa to guide the new drug through its testing period while the unconvinced were heard to mutter "It's murder" as they watched what he was doing.

The standard myth of penicillin gives the coming (or the mere threat) of World War II as the primary motivation for Florey and Chain's search for a new and more powerful antibacterial substance which could specifically be used for the treatment of war wounds. Both Florey and Chain have always denied this. Yet the coincidence of the start of the war and of the work that led to penicillin, plus the fact that penicillin achieved its impact on the world in the treatment of war wounds from the North African invasion onward have proved too powerful, too emotional, to permit the rest of us to believe the words of the men who really knew the truth because they had lived it.

Even the obituary of Lord Florey in the august pages of *Nature* on April 20, 1968, keeps it up: "With the outbreak of war in 1939 the potential importance of any substance capable of dealing with bacterial infection of wounds probably accentuated his interest in the field, but Florey was insistent that this was not just 'war work' but real science." So even a fellow scientist will not accept that it could have been "pure science" that produced a result so immediately important in the harsh world of reality as penicillin was to prove. The more dramatic accounts of the early writers about penicillin can be illustrated by extracts from Sokoloff's book:

> The idea that an antibacterial agent must exist was in the air. It was still not a very popular idea, it was still a stepchild of medical science. But more and more scientists turned to this problem. . . . The war was around the corner. The need for powerful antibacterial substances became of urgent practical importance. What of penicillin? It was only natural that this question should arise and be discussed at length in Florey's laboratory. It was decided to recultivate the mould discovered by Fleming, a culture of which was still alive.

Other accounts are quite definite that "the vital decision" to study penicillin was taken by Florey and Chain "under an elm tree." But the truth comes not merely from the memories of Florey and Chain. There is also documentary evidence that the myth is untrue.

Since the war was not the motive for Florey and Chain turning to penicillin, it was sheer luck, blind chance, that penicillin came into existence as a drug during the war years. What was not luck was the rapid rushing of penicillin into production. When chance provided the powerful antibacterial agent in the middle of a war, medical men and administrators on both sides of the Atlantic were quick enough to see what it meant and to manufacture the stuff in quantities and at a speed which would never have been possible in peacetime.

But the evidence from Oxford shows that it was also sheer

chance that made penicillin the first of the antibiotics. The
clues to the existence of other antibiotics were there in plenty
in 1938. Other scientists, notably René Dubos and Selman
Waksman in the U.S.A., were already beginning to look in this
direction. The luck of the Oxford men was that, for entirely the
wrong reasons, they chose to pick up the clue to the only
antibiotic which was not to be held up and delayed by problems of toxicity. And just as Florey and Chain have always
insisted that the war was not their motive, they have likewise
always insisted that their luck was fantastic.

To explain why it came about that penicillin was, for all practical purposes, discovered in Oxford, it is necessary to see how
the people involved got there.

Howard Walter Florey was an Australian and a brilliant
scholar. He was born in Adelaide, the capital of South Australia, on September 24, 1898; educated at St. Peter's Colle-
giate School, Adelaide, where he showed an early interest in
science, particularly in chemistry. Then he went on to Adelaide University where he qualified as a doctor. He came to
England in 1922 as a Rhodes scholar to Magdalen College,
Oxford, and at that time specialized in physiology. Following
a suggestion (probably from Sir Charles Sherrington) that he
should turn to pathology, he moved to Cambridge University
and started studying pathology there in 1924. A year in the
United States as a Rockefeller Foundation Fellow in 1925 was
followed by a spell of clinical experience at the London Hospital as a Freedom Research Fellow. He returned to Cambridge
again in 1929 and remained there until he was appointed
professor of pathology in Sheffield in 1931. The rapid rise and
career of a brilliant young man led to him being picked out,
largely by Sir Edward Mellanby, to be offered the chair at the
Sir William Dunn School of Pathology in Oxford in 1935.

Apart from its brilliance this was a thoroughly conventional
career up to this point. The only hints of significance for later
developments are three: Florey met the woman who was later

to be his first wife, Miss Ethel Reed, when they were both students at Adelaide; it was several years before they married and since Florey was not the sort of man who generated stories about significant incidents in his youth this is perhaps the first clue to his later consistency and strength of purpose. Then there is Florey's year in the U.S.A., during which he made many contacts and visited a number of different laboratories. But his principal activity there was a stay of several months at the University of Pennsylvania at Philadelphia where he made firm friends with Dr. A. Newton Richards. The third item of interest is that Florey became interested in the lysozyme discovered by Fleming in 1922, and while he was at Cambridge he started studying this substance. At first he worked on his own, then he joined with N.E. Goldsworthy. He kept up his interest in the subject and his work upon it when he went to Sheffield.

But the choice of Florey, at the age of only 37, to be professor of pathology at Oxford was a distinct act of policy. It was a quite deliberate act of choice, the bringing in of a physiologist, a man who was interested in the dynamics of living objects, a man with some clinical medical experience, to a subject which had in several universities become bogged down. At very nearly the same time another Australian physiologist was similarly appointed to the chair of pathology at University College Hospital in London. Florey's appointment to Oxford is described in his obituary in *Nature* as "a milestone in the history of pathology in Britain," and this is not because he later discovered penicillin, but in connection with the appointment of the other Australian in London: "Between them they laid down a new pattern for teaching and research in the pathology departments of Britain and the Commonwealth."

In Britain the precise forces behind such a movement are never as easily identifiable as they may be in the U.S.A. The Establishment, whoever they may be, decides that something must be done. This is not a formal decision of any particular committee or institution, it is a movement, usually of consensus opinion, among those in and around the field of action. In this case the moving spirit was Sir Edward Mellanby, a progressive and prominent figure in the world of medical research and secretary of the Medical Research Council. But the point is that Florey moved to Oxford backed by an influential movement of opinion, knowing that he was expected to inaugurate a new regime. His job was to build up a new type of pathology department. And that was exactly what he set about doing. He decided to go for what we know so well today as a multidisciplinary approach. Bacteriology, chemical pathology, and biochemistry were to be brought into one fold together, and the newest techniques of micromanipulation were to be used in pursuance of the physiological bias of Florey's own approach to pathology.

It was in Oxford—and perhaps in Oxford alone—in the Britain of those days, that the expertise that would be needed to solve the problems of penicillin had been drawn into one department, and this for reasons that had nothing to do with penicillin. Perhaps this was the greatest of all the strokes of fortune.

The career of Ernst Boris Chain was totally different. Born in Berlin in 1906, son of a Russian father (an industrialist in the chemical industry) and a German mother, Chain was one of the many German-Jewish scientists who had to flee when the Nazis came to power in 1933. By then he had obtained his medical qualifications and was starting to specialize in biochemistry. He came to England faced with having to start his career afresh. After working in London he managed to get started on some research work in the Institute of Biochemistry at Cambridge under Sir Frederick Gowland Hopkins, the man who established the importance of vitamins in diet. It was perhaps to Chain's advantage that he looked exactly what the English expect a young genius from the Continent to look like, in fact he looks like Einstein. He was also voluble and extrovert, a contrast to the reserved, very English-looking Florey.

Chain expected to go on to Canada or Australia to remake his life, so he was particularly delighted when he was offered a permanent post at Oxford by Florey. Gowland Hopkins had exerted himself considerably to get Chain such a job since he was much impressed by his work. And Chain's job was nothing less than to establish the study of biochemistry in the Sir William Dunn School of Pathology with a promise from Florey of a free hand for whatever personal research he wished. But Florey did suggest that lysozyme might be worth looking at.

Once Chain had joined Florey's staff at Oxford his work continued on the lines he had started at Cambridge. He examined the neurotoxins of some snake venoms and established that the substance that did the damage was an enzyme (a nucleotidase) which worked by knocking out one of the enzymes of the victim's body whose job was to perform a vital linking action in the control of the breathing system. In Chain's words: "Thus for the first time the mode of action of a natural toxin of protein nature could be explained in biochemical terms as that of an enzyme acting on a component of vital importance in the respiratory chain."

Enzymes are the specialist workmen of the body; each enzyme has a special task of ensuring that one of the many chemical reactions involved in living bodies is performed. There are thousands of such chemical changes involved in building cells, in converting food to energy, in breathing and converting oxygen to energy, in disposing of unwanted by-products. Some enzymes break down complicated molecules, such as incoming food, to simpler substances. Other enzymes have the job of linking together simple molecules into the long and complex molecules that make up the structures of the body. Enzymes are proteins, which means that they are molecules made up of the same basic units as the structural components of our bodies. These basic units are the twenty different amino-acids. Enzymes and all other proteins are long strings of these twenty basic building blocks. The order in which many hundreds of amino-acids are linked together defines the difference between one protein and another. But also, because of the mutual attractions and repulsions between the different types of amino-acid, the order also decides the way in which each of these long chains is twisted and folded together to make compact units.

It is generally held nowadays that an important factor in

deciding how enzymes work is the three-dimensional shape formed by this folding or twisting. Thus an enzyme may be shaped so that there is a cleft down one side. This cleft will enable the enzyme to fit over a protuberance in the shape of the protein that it is trying to break down. The strongest proof of this belief—that the shape of enzyme molecules matters in their way of working—has come from the elucidation of the full structure of lysozyme, and that has only been done within the last five years. None of this was known, and little was guessed at, in 1936, and Chain's work was one of the foundation stones of this modern science of enzyme chemistry.

When he had quickly finished his snake-venom work (no mean scientific achievement in itself) Chain turned to Florey's suggestion about lysozyme, and was given the assistance of a young American Rhodes scholar, Leslie A. Epstein. It will be remembered that Fleming had found lysozyme in 1922 in tears, in nasal mucus and in egg white, as well as in many other substances. He had also shown that it dissolved enormous numbers of the bacteria *Micrococcus lysodeikticus* in a dramatic manner. Chain declared in 1971: "The reason why Florey was interested in lysozyme was not so much its antibacterial power, which was of a very limited range, but the fact that, in addition to the sources just mentioned, it also occurred in duodenal secretions, and Florey thought at that time that it might play a role in the mechanisms of natural immunity and, in particular, could be involved in the pathogenesis of gastric ulcers." Chain was interested in lysozyme because it seemed to be an enzyme. Within a year he showed that it was in fact so, that its function was to break down a type of molecule called a polysaccharide, and that it attacked the micrococcus by breaking down its cell wall which contained such polysaccharide molecules.

This work was finished before the end of 1937, and in the process of writing it up for publication Chain started reading through the literature to discover comparable phenomena of the breaking-up, or lysis, of bacteria by natural substances. He found there were several recorded examples of one type of bacteria lysing another. But he found many more reports of cases where natural substances produced by bacteria, molds, streptomycetes and yeasts, prevented the growth and multiplication of bacteria without actually lysing them. He thus "stumbled more or less accidentally upon the subject of microbial antagonism." And he continues:

> However, next to nothing was known about the chemical or biological nature of the inhibitory substances and it seemed an interesting and rewarding field of exploration. After numerous discussions Florey and I decided jointly to undertake a systematic investigation of these antibacterial substances produced by micro-organisms from the chemical and biochemical as well as the biological point of view. . . . My part of this project was the isolation and study of the chemical and biochemical properties of these substances; Florey's the study of their biological properties.

Chain completed his extensive search of the scientific literature of bacterial antagonism early in 1938. In the process he came across Fleming's paper of 1929 which was one of the most striking accounts of bacterial inhibition anywhere in the literature.

A simple telling of the facts that led Florey and Chain toward penicillin can easily be made to seem like a logical progression of thought: Florey interested in lysozyme, which was Fleming's first antibacterial discovery; Florey puts Chain onto it; Chain solves lysozyme and they follow up the lead to Fleming's second antibacterial discovery. But in fact it was not like that. Florey was not interested in lysozyme as an antibacterial but as a physiological phenomenon. Chain only came across Fleming's second discovery in the course of a general search through the literature. There was not a drive toward penicillin, there was a much wider plan for a systematic scientific study of all microbial antagonisms.

But at this very time, the end of 1937 and the early months of 1938, there was an entirely different problem preying on Florey's mind: the quite unscientific matter of cash. The department was overdrawn at the bank by as much as £500, which seemed an enormous sum to the Oxford scientists of the time. Chain remembers distinctly an order coming from Florey forbidding him buying any more equipment or materials at all, not even a piece of glass tubing.

The first appeal for funds went to the Medical Research Council and was rejected. The business of yearly applications for small grants from the minor institutions known to British scientists appalled the scientists and seemed time-wasting. A long-term plan and major financial backing was what they needed, and Florey's thoughts turned to the Rockefeller Foundation which he knew from his year's study in America.

Florey first approached the Rockefeller Foundation late in 1938. The foundation made it known that if a proposal for a long-term program of research was put up it would receive favorable consideration as long as the proposal was of *a biochemical and not a medical nature* (author's italics).

There was the usual period of negotiation and visits by Rockefeller representatives to Oxford in the course of their trips to various European countries. Chain was asked by Florey to draw up a long-term biochemical program of research. He did so, making the systematic study of microbial antagonisms one half of it: "I included in this programme the project on antibacterial substances produced by micro-organisms, which could plausibly be expected to occupy us for quite a number of years."

The negotiations reached a climax on November 20, 1939 (two months after the war had begun, because these were gentlemanly transactions between a department at one of the world's greatest universities and one of the world's richest foundations). On that date Florey sent a formal proposal and request for support to the Rockefeller Foundation. Through the kindness of Professor Sir Ernst Chain I have obtained a copy of the full proposal, which I believe has never before been published. It opens with a letter from Florey to Dr. Warren Weaver:

> I had an opportunity of mentioning to Dr. Miller while he was visiting Oxford recently, that we had been preparing a statement

applying to the Trustees of the Rockefeller Foundation for a grant to enable us to carry out further biochemical investigations in this department. The statement was not ready at the time he was here, but Dr. Miller suggested that I should send it when completed to him in France to be transmitted for consideration through the usual channels. He thought however that as postal communication is now so uncertain that I should forward a copy direct to you in New York. I therefore enclose a copy of what I have sent to him.

So much for the urgent search for a cure for infected war wounds. It is positively reminiscent of Jane Austen: the war is not even mentioned but there is, instead, some uncertainty in postal communications.

The letter to Dr. H.M. Miller containing the official request for a grant is more detailed and makes it clear that the grant will be for the "enlargement and speeding up" of the biochemical research program. This program, Florey wrote

> has been continuously hampered by inadequate research funds and assistants, e.g., only one young technician has been available for four people. It has often taken months to get special pieces of apparatus owing to the necessity of approaching outside bodies, the trustees of which meet at long intervals, for relatively small sums of money. With the outbreak of war these material difficulties have not been lessened, but we are probably exceptionally fortunate in this department in that our essential research activities have been relatively little interfered with and our general research facilities remain as yet unimpaired.

Perhaps typical of Oxford: the nation at war but the essential researches "relatively little interfered with."

Florey then goes on to write of the importance he attaches to biochemistry and the importance he attaches to having Dr. Chain who has "a very great flair for the elucidation of enzyme as well as other biochemical problems." He ends with: "It may also be pointed out that the work proposed, in addition to its theoretical importance, may have practical value for therapeutic purposes." So there were Florey's priorities: work of theoretical biochemical importance first, but it *may* turn up something therapeutic.

The grant application then lists the six most important recent achievements of the department. First there is the construction (invention is implied) of a new type of microrespirometer which has been used to study the metabolism, the respiration and energy exchange of extremely small fragments of tissue containing very small numbers of cells. This was one of Florey's great personal interests, and he also compared the behavior of normal cells to cancer cells with this device. Then the work on snake venom and lysozyme is listed. Two more items, numbers four and five, do not concern this story at all. Finally it mentions what is called "spreading factor" and its relation to enzymes that break down the mucous membranes. Nine further pages are devoted to further details of this rather impressive three-year output of work and the papers published.

The nub of the application comes next, the program for several years of biochemical research. One half of this program—and only one half—involves penicillin. The crucial half of the program is "A chemical study of the phenomenon of bacterial antagonism with special consideration of bacteriolytic enzymes." The other half of the program was to be devoted to the study of the spreading factor mentioned above, which is also called mucinase.

This part of the application was the program drawn up by Chain at Florey's request. It began by summarizing bacterial antagonism and out of "many cases of bacterial antagonism" it chose three for specific mention: first *B. pyocyaneus*, which produces substances which destroy cholera, anthrax and diphtheria organisms; then *B. subtilis*, which produces something that stops the growth of pneumococci, streptococci and typhoid bacteria; the mold *Penicillium notatum* came only third, the last of the examples.

The letter of application explained why they thought the department should tackle the program:

The substances produced by bacteria in antagonism to each other act in a way similar to lysozyme, at least when they actually destroy other organisms. Lysozyme is an enzyme, which has been studied and has had its action elucidated in Oxford. It is likely that some of the other antagonistic substances are enzymes of the same group. They are, therefore, specific for bacteria, that is they attack only bacteria and are for this reason likely to be non-toxic to animal bodies. They seem therefore to possess great potentialities for therapeutic application. . . .

In view of the possibly great practical significance of antagonistic substances produced by bacteria against bacteria it is proposed to study systematically the chemical fundamentals of the phenomenon, with the aim of obtaining in purified state and suitable for intravenous injection, bacteriolytic and bactericidal substances against various kinds of pathogenic micro-organisms.

And then it reveals that they have already begun to try and purify the substances produced by the penicillium mold *and* the pyocyaneus bacilli. The remainder of Chain's paper contains details of the proposed work on mucinase. There is also a reassurance that Professor Florey and Professor Gardner will be available to carry out the biological work and animal experiments.

But plainly, from Chain's outline, we see that he had the same priorities as Florey. The work was to be a broad and systematic study of a wide range of phenomena, getting down to the chemical fundamentals before preparing anything practical. Within about a year of this application the authors were to be more interested in getting enough penicillin to start treating patients than with the chemical fundamentals.

It tells much about the times and the conditions in which these men worked, to give some of the details of proposed expenditure which Florey provided for the Rockefeller Foundation. He wanted two more technicians, total salary £320 a year; a mechanic at £250. Even the fully qualified biochemist would only get £600 a year. The equipment included a fast centrifuge at £150, but he also wanted to buy a volt-amp meter at £5 and an ice-crushing machine for £10. The dramatic tellers of the story of penicillin have much to say about the sylvan beauties of Florey's laboratories on the edge of Oxford's parks, where the university cricket team plays its matches. But they say nothing about "progress towards penicillin" needing a "small Latapie mincer" costing £15.

Rockefeller, however, felt there was even a need for a "large Latapie mincer" costing £53. The foundation offered $5000 a year for five years, which Chain says "seemed royal generosity to us."

The picture of a race to produce an antibacterial drug to save soldiers' lives is strongly denied by Professor Chain. He told me: "There was no race, not a race to produce penicillin for the war, not a race against anyone else. If anyone else had been working on the subject I would not have been interested. It was getting the whole field opened up that interested me, and the Rockefeller grant was the most important thing for that. We happened to go for penicillin because we had a culture growing at the school."

HOW IT WAS DONE

The work at Oxford set off on the wrong foot. With the two major scientific successes of snake venom and lysozyme just behind them, both Chain and Florey thought that the antibacterial substances were almost certainly enzymes. And they had good reason for believing that penicillin, too, was an enzyme.

Exactly thirty years after the event Chain told a symposium on penicillin:

> When I saw Fleming's paper for the first time I thought that Fleming had discovered a sort of mould lysozyme, which, in contrast to egg-white lysozyme, acted on a wide range of Gram-positive pathogenic bacteria. I further thought that in all probability the cell walls of all these pathogenic bacteria whose growth was inhibited by the mould lysozyme contained a common substrate on which the supposed enzyme acted and that it would be worthwhile to try and isolate and characterise the hypothetical common substrate. For this purpose it would, of course, be necessary to purify the supposed enzyme, but I did not foresee any undue difficulties with this task for which I was well prepared from my previous research experience. At that time I was actually more

interested in studying the substrate of the supposed enzyme than the enzyme itself. My belief that we were dealing with an enzyme was strengthened by a paper from the laboratory of Raistrick and collaborators which had appeared in 1932 and in which the observations on the instability of penicillin already recorded by Fleming were confirmed and extended. These authors found that on extracting the acidified penicillin-containing culture fluid the active principle disappeared from the aqueous phase [i.e., passed out of the watery solution into the ether] but could not be recovered after evaporation of the ether. I interpreted these results as indicating surface denaturation of the supposed active protein by ether, such as occurs readily with lysozyme. My working hypothesis proved completely erroneous as my first experiments were to prove very soon.

But Chain was right in one respect, as it turned out years later. Penicillin, although it was not an enzyme, did act on a particular substance which is common to the cell walls of all the bacteria that are attacked by penicillin. However, it *does not* break down a substance in the cell wall, as lysozyme does; penicillin *prevents* the particular substrate from being successfully built into the cell wall.

The systematic study of bacterial antagonism planned by Florey and Chain had begun on a very small scale before the Rockefeller grant made a large scale progress possible. In early 1939 they had decided to start with three different substances: the pyocyanase produced by *B. pyocyaneus,* the penicillin noted by Fleming and the substances produced by the large group of fungi called actinomycetes. The work on these last never got started at all at Oxford, though they were later to provide famous antibiotics for other workers.

Rapid progress was first made with pyocyanase, which had also been studied in Germany and which had even been used in some crude clinical work on the Continent. Soon Chain had extracted two substances from this organism, but the very first animal experiments showed them to be extremely toxic. Nevertheless, work on the pyocyanase went on in parallel with work on penicillin.

The Sir William Dunn School of Pathology possessed examples of Fleming's strain of *Penicillium notatum*. This was a strange coincidence, because Chain certainly discovered Fleming's work by reading the literature and not by any knowledge of previous work at Oxford. But the fact that the mold was in their possession undoubtedly led them to choose penicillin as one of the starting points of their grand survey of microbial antagonism. The mold was in Oxford because Florey's predecessor, Professor Georges Dreyer, had been working on bacteriophage at the time of Fleming's original observation and had wondered whether penicillin was an example of bacteriophage. Bacteriophage, now known to exist in many different strains and types, is a virus which infects and kills bacteria. As soon as Dreyer found out that penicillin was nothing like bacteriophage he stopped studying it. There is a story about Chain in his first days at Oxford having bumped into a laboratory assistant carrying a tray of flasks along the corridor and asking what was in the flasks. When he had read Fleming's paper he remembered the incident in the corridor and went to the laboratory of Miss Margaret Campbell-Renton, who had been Dreyer's assistant, and got the mold from her.

Chain took from Raistrick's work the knowledge that the mold could be grown on the synthetic, and easily managed, Czapek-Dox medium, modified by the addition of glucose. The early months of 1939 were mostly taken up with learning how to grow the penicillium mold so that it would produce penicillin. Chain met the same problems of variability in mold performance, and rapid mutation in the mold strains, that had discouraged Dr. Paine in Sheffield. The work on pyocyanase proceeded more rapidly and smoothly up to the time of the 1939 summer holidays and beyond. Chain took his holiday in Belgium and had to come hurrying back to return before the war broke out.

It was the outbreak of the war that brought Norman Heatley (Dr. N.G. Heatley) into the story. He had also been recruited by Florey, and lured from Cambridge to Oxford. Heatley's speciality was with microtechniques. He was one of the pioneers and marvelously skilled at producing new devices and working them; he came to Oxford for the microrespirometer work. Heatley was, in the summer of 1939, planning to change his job and have a year's experience in the laboratories of Copenhagen University. He was expecting to sail to Denmark on September 12 and he had his bags packed when the trip had to be called off because of the war. So he stayed in Oxford and was immediately asked by Florey to help Chain. He started work early in 1940 and took over the growing of the mold and the basic testing and measuring of strengths and potencies of penicillin.

Heatley is undoubtedly one of the most engaging characters in the entire penicillin story. In contrast to the strength of Florey the Australian, and the ebullience of Chain, the Russo-German Jew, the gentle unassuming Heatley almost disappears from sight. He is completely English middle class, with a conventional career through public school to Cambridge. He still works in the Sir William Dunn School at Oxford, and his outstanding quality is still his shyness. There is an obituary of Lord Florey in the *Journal of General Microbiology* (1970) written entirely in that reserved third-person style favored by British scientists; it contains the following remark about Heatley and his work in the early days of producing penicillin: "his forte was improvisation, a quality normally of little value to a research worker, though it proved useful under the wartime conditions of restriction and shortage." It is only when the reader comes to the end of this obituary notice that he may find that the author is N.G. Heatley.

With Heatley taking over the growing of the mold and the testing of the strength of penicillin against standard preparations of microbes in Petri dishes, Chain was able to concentrate on the chemical work of purifying and isolating the substance. He immediately got a shock. The penicillin was not an enzyme at all. The active substance passed easily through cellophane filters and therefore could not possibly be a large molecule of the enzyme type. It must be a small and comparatively simple molecule. Chain comments:

I was at first disappointed with the finding, for my beautiful working hypothesis dissolved into thin air, yet the fact of the instability of penicillin remained and became even more puzzling as it could not be explained on the basis of being a protein. There was at that time no other antibacterial with that degree of instability known, and it became very interesting to find out which structural features were responsible for the instability. It was clear that we were dealing with a chemically very unusual substance and thus it was of obvious interest to continue with the work. Only the nature of our problem had changed: instead of studying the isolation and mode of action of an enzyme with strong antibacterial properties, our task was now the elucidation of the structure of a low molecular substance which combined high antibacterial power with great chemical instability.

It was the instability of penicillin, its habit of just disappearing, that had baffled Fleming and his assistants; it was instability that caused Raistrick to lose interest; it was instability that attracted Chain, because it made him think he had an enzyme to deal with. When it turned out that penicillin was not an enzyme the instability became so extraordinary that it piqued Chain's curiosity and he just had to pursue penicillin out of true scientific interest.

Chain proceeded with the usual methods for extracting penicillin from the mold juice: moving the penicillin from water into solvent and back to water hoping to leave impurities behind at each move. But he began from a slightly different angle. Because he was fascinated by the very instability of the substance, he started by testing its stability at different pH levels. This showed that it was only stable between pH 5 and pH 8, that is, in a very narrow range near to neutrality between acid and alkali. Yet the methods used to move the penicillin from one solvent to another involved acidities very close to the limits of the range. Chain found that keeping the whole mixture at 0° C slowed down the rate of inactivation of the penicillin and by careful adjustment of acidity levels, and frequent returns to neutral (pH 7) by the addition of alkali, he could advance one stage beyond Raistrick's ether stage and could get most of the activity back into water. But he still could not dry out or crystallize this solution to dryness without destroying the penicillin.

Eventually he tried freeze-drying. This process, quite familiar to us in the 1970s as a common method of preserving food, particularly vegetables, had been known as a laboratory method for many years before Chain tried it on penicillin. However, just before 1940 it had been introduced on a larger scale at Cambridge for the drying of blood serum. At any rate, it provided Chain with a little dry brown powder. Then came two big surprises.

In the routine testing of this dry brown powder, to see whether the penicillin had been destroyed or had survived, it suddenly turned out that the powder had strong antibacterial action even at dilutions of 1 in 10^6. They were faced, in fact, with a substance that could stop bacteria growing when there was only one drop of it in a million drops of water. It was twenty times more active than the most powerful sulphonamide then known.

Still as a matter of routine "and without any optimistic expectations" (Chain's words) the powder was tested on mice to see if it was toxic. To the amazement of them all there was no damage to mice even when they were given the enormous dose (enormous to a mouse at least) of twenty milligrams.

Florey and Gardner happened to be away the day this test was done. Chain had the work performed by Dr. John M. Barnes, who was not officially in Chain's unit but worked directly upstairs. Florey was so astounded when he heard about the toxicity test that he immediately did it again himself, though it was by no means easy for Chain to produce another twenty milligrams of the powder. Once again the substance proved to be non-toxic.

These mice which had survived the toxicity tests showed an odd thing. Their urine turned the same dark brown color as the penicillin preparations. The urine was examined and was found to be highly active against bacteria. Chain remembers: "From this we concluded that penicillin passed through the body of the mouse without loss of activity and that it was therefore probable that it would display its antibacterial activity in the body fluids. This looked promising from the chemotherapeutic point of view."

There is no doubt that this is the critical point in the history of penicillin. This was the moment the vision of an antibiotic really entered men's minds, a naturally produced substance which could be safely put inside living bodies where it would circulate inside the system and defeat infections from within. (Incidentally, if penicillin had been an enzyme it could never have had these therapeutic possibilities since a foreign protein cannot be introduced into the body without causing violent immunological reactions.) And it was just here that the breakthrough in thinking worked by the sulphonamides became effective, for the sulpha drugs had prepared scientists to think of chemicals working inside the body rather than the external "antiseptic" applications tried by Fleming and Dr. Paine.

So the crucial experiment to see whether penicillin was a practical chemotherapeutic agent, the experiment that Fleming and Raistrick had failed to perform, was set up. At this stage of the penicillin story precise dates begin to be known.

Penicillin, the first antibiotic, began its curative work on May 25, 1940. This was a Saturday, and even in wartime Saturday is part of the British weekend, so the excitement must have been intense. But it was probably still mostly scientific excitement, and not yet the hunt for a cure for infected war-wounds. Eight white mice were each given lethal doses of streptococci in the stomach cavity. An hour after this two of them were given single doses of ten milligrams of penicillin (or, more accurately, of Chain's powder in distilled water). Two more mice were given doses of five milligrams of penicillin, and these two mice were given repeats of the same dose three times at two-hour intervals. These mice also received a final five milligram dose of penicillin four hours later. The laboratory notebook records in bald prose what happened: "All four control mice which had received no penicillin died between thirteen and sixteen and a half hours after infection, when the treated mice were all alive and well. The treated mice receiving the smaller dose died after two and six days, the other two surviving without sign of sickness."

Florey himself performed this experiment. When he left the laboratory on that Saturday evening he already had a strong hint from the mice that penicillin was going to prove exciting: the control mice were already looking ill and the treated mice appeared quite well. Heatley would not even leave the experiment and stayed with it most of the night, in fact until the four control mice had died. This is why the exact timings of death—"between thirteen and sixteen and a half hours after infection" have been so precisely noted. When he left at 3:45 a.m. on the morning of Sunday, May 26, the two mice treated with the smaller dose were beginning to look seedy, with their coats fluffing out, but the other two, with the big doses, were quite well. Penicillin had, in fact, proved itself already by providing some measure of protection against the massive dose of germs. Heatley cycled home in the early hours of that May morning and he still remembers being stopped by a keen Home Guard and having to explain his presence in the Oxford streets at such an unearthly hour.

After a few hours of sleep Heatley returned to the laboratory to look at the progress of the experiment again. He found Florey and Chain already there looking at the four dead controls and the four live treated mice. Chain—obviously excited, slightly flushed, but strangely silent—replied mostly by shrugging his shoulders. Florey committed himself to saying, "It looks very promising." But his actions spoke louder than words. Heatley wrote in his obituary of Florey: "It is typical of Florey's drive that within twenty-six hours of the *beginning* of the experiment—long before it was completed—plans had been laid for increased production of penicillin by all means possible."

The big problem, which none of them realized in those moments of excitement and delight, was that the stuff with which they had treated the mice was hardly "penicillin" at all. It was ninety-nine percent impurities and only one percent pure penicillin.

There were at least three other people directly involved in

these mouse experiments that proved the power and usefulness of penicillin. These were Professor Arthur D. Gardner
and his colleague Miss Jean Orr-Ewing, and Florey's technical
assistant Mr. James Kent. Also by this time Dr. (now Professor)
Edward P. Abraham had moved across from the nearby Dyson
Perrins Chemistry Laboratory to help Chain with the chemical
work.

It took only three months from the May 25 experiment on
eight mice to prove that penicillin was really going to be a
major chemotherapeutic agent, and to present the news to the
world. It was on August 24, 1940, that Florey, Chain and their
collaborators (Heatley, Gardner, Orr-Ewing, Margaret Jennings and Gordon Sanders) published in the *Lancet* the first of
their world-shaking papers, "Penicillin as a chemotherapeutic
agent."

On the morning of the mouse experiments, Sunday, May
26, 1940, Florey decided immediately to increase production
of penicillin. Chain explained in 1971 why this decision was
taken:

> This experiment was in essence the demonstration of the chemo-
> therapeutic effect of penicillin. Everything that followed was,
> more or less, in the nature of routine operations. It was evidently
> necessary to extend the chemotherapeutic experiments to other
> pathogens sensitive to penicillin [other germs must be tested]—
> this needed more material. It was necessary to study the phar-
> macological properties of penicillin—this needed still more
> material. Finally it was more necessary than ever to press on with
> the chemical studies—this needed yet considerably more
> material.

The paper in the *Lancet* says little or nothing about these
efforts to get more material and purer material. It simply emphasizes, twice, that the preliminary experiments have all been
done with impure material which makes the effects reported
even more impressive. The paper opens with a sober recital of
the motives and origins of the penicillin investigation.

> In recent years interest in chemotherapeutic effects has been al-
> most exclusively focussed on the sulphonamides and their deriva-

tives. There are, however, other possibilities notably those connected with naturally occurring substances. . . . Following the work on lysozyme in this laboratory it occurred to two of us (E.C. and H.W.F.) that it would be profitable to conduct a systematic investigation of the chemical and biological properties of the antibacterial substances produced by bacteria and moulds.

The work of Fleming, Raistrick and Reid are duly noted, for none of the other work had been published, but the failure to isolate penicillin was recorded. With considerable modesty the next paragraph says: "During the last year methods have been devised here for obtaining a considerable yield of penicillin and for rapid assay of its inhibitory power. From the culture medium a brown powder has been obtained which is freely soluble in water. It and its solution are stable for a considerable time and though it is not a pure substance its antibacterial activity is very great."

Slowly the paper plows through the many toxicity tests, including tests on rats and cats, which the group had performed that summer. Then the tests on the pharmacological activity of the substance, its effect on breathing, heart rate and blood pressure; its reappearance in the urine; some slight signs of kidney damage in rats, but no long-term damage to blood cells and particularly no damage to white cells (leucocytes). Then further tests on the antibacterial action in vitro (that is, what germs it killed in Petri dishes). "Penicillin is not immediately bactericidal but seems to interfere with multiplication"; and again one wonders why no one before Professor Hare in the late 1960s queried Fleming's original observation which said that penicillin *did* kill germs in the Petri dish. A number of germs affected by penicillin were added to Fleming's original list, notably members of the *Clostridia* family of microbes, some of which are responsible for causing gas gangrene, the most feared infection of wounds.

At last we come to what it was really all about, the "therapeutic effects." Five big experiments are reported each involving between forty-eight and seventy-five mice. Three important dangerous germs were tested: a staphylococcus, a streptococcus and a clostridium. In every case those mice treated with penicillin were shown to have been given protection against the germs. In every experiment but one all the control mice died, and only four survivors are recorded in the remaining experiment. In all cases a significant number of treated mice survived and in the most impressive example twenty-four out of twenty-five infected animals were saved by penicillin.

The paper ends with a very firm conclusion: "The results are clear cut, and show that penicillin is active in vivo against at least three of the organisms inhibited in vitro. It would seem a reasonable hope that all organisms inhibited in high dilution in vitro will be found to be dealt with in vivo. Penicillin does not appear to be related to any chemotherapeutic substance at present in use, and is particularly remarkable for its activity against the anaerobic organisms associated with gas gangrene."

The original experiments on the eight mice, the experiment of May 25, is not included in the paper, and our only record of that crucial weekend comes from memories and Heatley's laboratory notes.

It all amounts to a very impressive output for less than three months' work. But those three months, from May to August 1940, had also been the time for what seemed even more impressive results by the German armies in Europe. It was only now that the war fever really affected the Oxford scientists. It was at this stage that those in the know at the Sir William Dunn School—Florey, Chain, Heatley, Gardner and young Dr. Margaret A. Jennings who had handled the mice and done much of the injecting during the big experiments— smeared the linings of their clothes with the mold. If the Germans invaded someone would get away to somewhere, Canada or the U.S.A. perhaps, and be able to isolate spores of the mold from their clothing and carry on the work. The mold stain was a dreary brown and would not be noticed.

Chapter 11
HEROIC DAYS

THESE WERE THE HEROIC DAYS of penicillin, the last half of 1940 and the first months of 1941. There were just eight scientists, (Florey, Chain, Gardner, Heatley, Jennings, Sanders and Abraham and Orr-Ewing), assisted by the faithful J. Kent and never more than a couple of technicians. This was the "Oxford team."

There is a problem about this Oxford team though. The members of it do not remember it as being a team at all, at least not in the sense that we nowadays build up a scientific team. At least six of the members were not working fulltime on penicillin. It was a much more subtle thing than a team; it was a collection of specialists each doing his own job when called upon to do so. The linking factor was Florey. It was he who called it a team (after it had finished its work) and the conclusion must be that he used the phrase "a team effort" in a rather loose cliché-ish way to avoid having to take all the credit himself. It is this cliché that has stuck.

Heatley, for instance, makes it quite clear that the claim for a team effort was Florey's own.

Florey was once maliciously described as a physiologist who happened to have in his department the right people to work through the project. He would have been the first to disclaim expert knowledge in, for example, chemistry or bacteriology, but those who knew him know also what shrewd comments and suggestions he could make in fields other than his own. He repeatedly stressed that the outcome was the product of a team and was scrupulous in giving all possible credit to the other members of it. But he had prepared the ground at Oxford by building up during previous years a laboratory intentionally staffed with workers trained in a variety of disciplines. This was a logical extension of his conviction—shared by few others when he came to Oxford in 1935— that advances in medicine were most likely to spring from rigorous experiment in the basic medical sciences.

At the purely practical level his own contributions were substantial and crucial. . . . A colleague remarked of this phase that "not an experiment was wasted, and these early animal experiments provided a firm basis for planning human therapy. Without them, the results from the treatment of the first half dozen human patients might well have been inconclusive instead of clear-cut, with who knows what frustration and delay in the introduction of penicillin into medicine."

Important as this work was, it is in his other role, as leader of the team, that Florey was irreplaceable. One remembers his humour, his infectious enthusiasm and his genial and constructive cynicism. Certain decisions he made boldly and swiftly on his own initiative and responsibility; but in general he constantly consulted his colleagues and allowed them virtually complete freedom to pursue their own branch of the work as they thought best —or rather as they thought best after discussion with him or with another colleague. *There were few meetings of "the team" as such* [author's stress], but many informal discussions with individuals or small groups enabled Florey constantly to reassess the course of the work and to suggest revisions of the immediate programme. In retrospect, though there were many disappointments and failures, there were few if any occasions when some remedy or alternative approach could not be suggested. **How remarkably** effective was his firm but unobtrusive leadership is shown by the fact that the first clinical trials were completed after no more than eighteen months of sustained work.

Professor Chain and Professor Charles Fletcher, who joined the team to perform the first applications of penicillin to human patients, have both confirmed that Heatley's view of "a group of specialists" is closer to the truth than our usual idea of a team.

Florey himself published a great deal of purely scientific work about penicillin and other antibiotics. All his papers had the virtue of clarity. He spoke well and clearly. But he was reserved, especially about personal matters; he did not let his feelings show, at least outside the world of his scientific colleagues. He was not the sort of man who generated legends about himself, and he would have hated to think that any legends existed about him. A single sentence from Heatley's obituary of the man makes the point: "Naturally no hint was permitted in any publication from Florey's department of the crucial part he played in encouraging and inspiring his colleagues, in directing the project so effectively and unobtrusively, or in the clear-cut elegance of his own laboratory work." The scientific publications from the Oxford workers, the historic papers announcing in 1940 and 1941, first that penicillin was a chemotherapeutic agent and then that it had cured human beings, carry the names of the authors strictly in alphabetic order. Florey appears second in the first paper, after Chain, and fourth in the second paper, after Abraham, Chain and Fletcher. There is no indication that he is the professor or in any way leader of the team.

The fact that the team was a group of specialists makes it impossible to construct a coherent and consecutive narrative of their work. Many different things were being done at the same time. The attempts to increase production of penicillin started directly after the May 25 experiment and continued into 1941. At the same time the chemical work of Chain and Abraham to achieve greater purification continued. The biological testing by Gardner and Florey likewise went ahead and developed into the first clinical tests on humans at a rate determined by progress in the first two fields. And at the same time Florey was beginning to explore the possibility of getting commercial firms in Britain to take up the manufacture and testing of this very promising new substance. His rebuffs by industry placed an even greater pressure on "the production department"; in any case it was unprecedented for a university laboratory, and in Oxford of all places, to have a production department.

However, the production department worked on, and, as they produced material, Florey and Gardner repeated and confirmed the mouse tests reported in the August paper, extending them to show that penicillin worked against yet other types of microbes in infected mice. But it was the beginning of 1941 before they dared to try anything on a human being. The first human was a volunteer, an unnamed woman who was dying of cancer. There was no attempt at a cure, it was simply to see what happened when a human was injected with penicillin.

The injection was given by Dr. Charles Fletcher, then a young medical registrar, working as a Nuffield research student. He injected 100 milligrams of penicillin into the patient. This was a carefully calculated dose. Twenty milligrams had proved harmless to a mouse, and since in Florey's words, "a man is 3000 times the size of a mouse," 100 milligrams should certainly have been safe for a human. Yet the patient showed an immediate reaction of the type known to doctors as rigor. This is rather like having flu; there is shivering and a sudden high temperature. This was bad news and they all knew what it meant. There must still be impurities in the penicillin and these impurities were pyrogens, fever producers. The impurities could be proteins left over from the mold itself or its metabolism, or even some effect of the glucose added to the original medium.

The experiment was performed on January 17, 1941. Since it was an historic occasion it is appropriate that we should know the exact date. For a change, it is the historian who has this time a bit of luck in the penicillin story. It was some years after the experiment that Lady Florey started to inquire about the exact date. Naturally, she asked Charles Fletcher and he promised to look up his clinical notes. But among all the material on penicillin trials there was no note of the date. So he suggested that they should look up the patient's case notes at the hospital. (The patient had, of course, been dead for some years by then.) But even more strangely, or perhaps because they had all been so excited, there was no record in the case notes of the penicillin injection. But then Fletcher remembered the rigor and looked at the patient's temperature chart, which as usual had been kept at the foot of the bed until filed with the case notes. And there, sure enough was the "spike" of sudden fever which the nurses had duly filled in on the chart. And so the date was found.

The real worry to the Oxford men was the outside possibility that it might have been penicillin itself that had caused the toxic reaction in the human. Fortunately, Abraham had already started chromatography tests on the penicillin powder. (Chromatography is a technique in which any complex of substances can be split up into its component parts by letting a solution of the original run down a sheet or column of some absorbent material. The different components of the original complex run at slightly different speeds because the molecules are slightly different in size and weight and solubility. Eventually, each component can be found in a separate band or patch according to the material on which the chromatography has been performed.) Abraham split up the penicillin powder by letting a solution of the powder run through a long glass tube containing alumina powder. Each component separated by the column of powder was then tested to see which one contained the activity of penicillin. The penicillin-containing fraction of the original powder was then tested on rabbits by Florey and found to be free from pyrogens. This was "to everyone's relief," according to Heatley and it may be assumed that this is an understatement.

We know now that the original penicillin powder contained, in fact, some thirty different substances. The extra purification by chromatography became a routine part of the production of penicillin in the laboratory from this stage onward. And we know that the penicillin they were about to use in attempts to cure human patients still carried with it several impurities, and it was their luck that these impurities were not toxic.

Various members of the Oxford team and other people on the staff of the Sir William Dunn School were the next volunteers. Fletcher gave them penicillin by a variety of routes, and the rabbit experiment was confirmed; they now had a substance that was non-toxic even to humans. These volunteers had to give blood and urine samples and it was duly established what levels of penicillin in the blood followed different sizes of dose, and what amount of penicillin was excreted through the kidneys. There was also at this stage a certain amount of application of penicillin to various minor external infections by members of the group, and Florey tried treating a stye from which he was suffering.

It took another month after the first injection of penicillin into a human to complete the purification trials and to amass enough material to consider treating a patient with a serious infection. The penicillin was now coming off Heatley's production line as very small quantities of yellowish powder and was stored in the refrigerator. The application to human treatment was entirely different from the way a new drug is brought into use nowadays. Florey had decided that the best way to administer the drug at first would be by continuous intravenous infusion, a drip system. There was no question of penicillin being administered by mouth, since Chain's showing of its instability to acid promised that any penicillin administered by mouth would be immediately destroyed by the acids of the stomach before it got any chance to work into the patient's system. What finally happened was no careful accumulation of enough penicillin to enable them to treat a case properly. They came across a case so desperate that it seemed, firstly, worth taking the risk of trying out a completely untested drug, and so desperate, secondly, that anything was worth trying.

It was an Oxford policeman, Albert Alexander, who had originally suffered from nothing worse than a scratch on the face from a rose bush, a scratch near the corner of his mouth. Unfortunately the slight wound became infected with *Staphylococcus aureus* and as the weeks passed a streptococcal infection was added. He was duly admitted to the Radcliffe Infirmary, but nothing could stop the infection. After two months of treatment the doctors despaired of the man. They had treated him with the latest of the sulphonamides, sulphapyridine, and were draining the worst of his abscesses artificially. He had by now lost one eye and his lungs were beginning to be affected.

On February 12, 1941, Dr. Fletcher started treating him with penicillin. A first dose of 400 milligrams was followed by an intravenous drip feeding him 100 milligrams of the drug every three hours. The effect was striking; within twenty-four hours the policeman was plainly very much better. The case notes record: "Striking improvement after total of 800 milligrams penicillin in twenty-four hours." The fever started to go down, the abscesses ceased to discharge, the running from the eye stopped. The next day the penicillin treatment continued, and so did the improvement. But the penicillin was being used up at the rate of one gram every twenty-four hours and it was already becoming doubtful whether they would have enough.

Dr. Fletcher started collecting the policeman's urine and taking it back to the laboratory to have the penicillin extracted from it. Three days later the policeman was receiving the same penicillin that he had received on the first day, after it had been reprocessed from his urine. The patient was also given a large blood transfusion, and his improvement continued as long as the penicillin held out. He was even eating by the fourth day and the fever had totally disappeared. But by the fifth day they had given him four and a half grams of penicillin, their whole stock and what had been recovered from the urine. They had no more to give. For ten days the policeman seemed to hold his own against the half-cured infection, but then the staphylococci and streptococci got the upper hand and on March 15 the patient died. What Florey called "this forlorn case" had, in fact, convinced him and his colleagues of the extraordinary value of penicillin. This in one way made it worse for them that they had failed, when they were sure they had had enough of the drug. The result was, of course, even greater demand for supplies. And this time they waited until they knew they had enough before starting treatment.

But they also eased the strain on the supplies of penicillin by deciding to treat children. Children are, as one might say, halfway between a man and a mouse, at least in size. Treating children would require less penicillin than treating full-sized adults. But they also knew from the case of the policeman that the penicillin was excreted so quickly that the task of trying to keep an adequate level of penicillin in the blood was "like trying to fill a bath with the plug out." The graphic but simple description is recognizably Florey's.

Five more patients were treated in the three months following the tragedy of the policeman, and four of these were children. All were cured of their infections. But more than that, to those involved, the effect of penicillin seemed miraculous. This is a word that is easily used by most of us; for a scientist or a doctor to bring himself to use it is much harder. Yet the eminently quiet and sober Heatley allows himself: "it must suffice to record here that the response to penicillin was considered almost miraculous." And it is fairly easy to find doctors who remember the first cases they saw cured by penicillin, and the word crops up again and again. No one really means miraculous in a strict sense, but the results were so surprising to those who had worked in the days before penicillin became available that this was the word with which they reacted.

The most severely afflicted of the four children treated at this time was suffering from a condition known as cavernous sinus thrombosis, an infected blood clot in the brain. This condition at that time was considered invariably fatal. Furthermore, it produced a most distressing appearance, with the eyes apparently bursting out of the head. The boy was not even conscious when the treatment with penicillin started, but within a few days he was clearly better, the distressing symptoms had disappeared, and within a couple of weeks the child was playing with his toys, eating normally and apparently quite recovered. Suddenly he died. The post-mortem showed that death was due to the rupture of an artery in the head, an artery weakened by the pressure of the earlier infection. The death was, of course, a tragedy in itself, but the cold, medical and objective fact was that the post-mortem allowed it to be shown quite clearly that all trace of infection had been wiped out and that the internal lesions had completely cleared up. In fact this post-mortem enabled the medical scientists to show conclusively that penicillin had cured the infection, whereas with those cases where the patient survived it could always have been argued that the body's natural defenses had at last won their battle, or that some other fortuitous happening had caused the recovery.

In the cases of two other children treated at this time, an infection of the bone of the hip was cured in a fifteen-year-old boy, and a lung infection was dealt with in another child. In the report on the boy with the hip infection Florey wrote: "Penicillin therapy was followed by a great improvement in the patient's general condition, in spite of the dose being insufficient to maintain a detectable concentration of penicillin continuously in the blood." The only adult in this little group of five cases was treated for a carbuncle, which was four inches across at the start of treatment; it was healing within four days and the patient was discharged in twelve days.

Such few results would not be considered as proving anything nowadays. But it was the quality of the effects, the "miraculous" results, that impressed those who were doing the work. Florey certainly felt that the clinical results were good enough for further action to be taken. A further paper was published in the *Lancet* describing the human cures. This paper is referred to as "Abraham 1941" from the first name in the list of authors. Chain, Fletcher, Florey, Gardner, Heatley and Jennings were the other names. The title was an essay in understatement: "Further observations on penicillin." The important thing is that at this stage the Oxford men were quite convinced that they had one of the most remarkable medical discoveries of all time on their hands.

We can look back now and agree that they were right to be convinced. But Professor Stewart has some sobering words:

> The results were convincing, each in a different way, and the absence of toxicity was almost as impressive as the rapid therapeutic effect. In the present day [1965 when Stewart wrote], when a clinical trial is becoming an exercise in statistics and bureaucracy, there is irony in the reflection that the massive efforts which followed were based upon a few toxicity tests in rodents and upon a clinical trial in six selected subjects, two of whom died. Had the toxicity tests been extended to guinea-pigs, penicillin might have been rejected; had current regulations been in force, it would have been ineligible for submission.

Bold decisions made on small quantities of fairly convincing evidence; decisions made about a substance which seemed to have curative powers never before witnessed by man; these decisions we now see to have been broadly correct every time. These were, indeed, heroic days. But the labor and effort of a very small number of people—a few girls, a couple of technicians and Heatley—in steadily increasing production of penicillin were an absolutely necessary condition for the more dramatic efforts of the biologists, physiologists and doctors. There was a good deal of heroic improvisation in the production department, too, involving the use of such diverse materials as old bookshelves from the Bodleian library, bedpans, and glass bottles originally designed to carry concentrated soft drinks.

Heatley, foiled by the outbreak of war of his opportunity to work in Denmark, had been given the task, first to grow the mold, then to work out methods of testing and measuring, and finally, by a natural process, he graduated to production. Growing the mold had been started on the Czapek-Dox medium, and the first thing was to try variations of the medium. Glutamine, glycerol peptone, thyoglycollic acid, were all added to no great benefit. Variations in temperature, acidity, methods of inoculating the medium with mold spores, likewise gave no improvement. Household foods like Marmite were tried, and they even went back at one stage to broths made of horse or cow meat. The only thing that really did any good was boiled brewers' yeast. The boiled yeast, added to the Czapek-Dox medium, did show a definite increase in the rate of growth of the mold and in the amount of penicillin produced, and this medium continued to be used throughout the Oxford work. There was the one little oddity: it did not seem to matter how much of the yeast they put in; ten percent or only a quarter of that amount produced exactly the same improvement in yield.

Heatley's next big step forward was to work out a way in which the medium containing the penicillin could be harvested from under a fully grown mold without disturbing the mold. By replacing the medium with a fresh solution the long delay of waiting several days for a fresh growth of mold could be avoided, because the fully grown mold would carry on producing penicillin as long as it was provided with fresh medium. Heatley devised a simple hand-held device which fed in sterile compressed air underneath the mold as the penicillin-containing medium was drawn off. Then an inflow of fresh medium drove out the air and the mold was left sitting on top of a flaskful of new medium. He eventually persuaded the molds to grow on as many as twelve consecutive refills of fresh medium, and, since the saving of growing time was equivalent to saving one third of production time each round, this made a considerable improvement in method. It further saved a great deal of glass washing and sterilization, and was used for at least two years at Oxford. Eventually, however, a contaminant mold became so well established in the buildings and spoiled so many cultures that the system had to be abandoned.

The "cup-plate assay" was being developed at this time, too. In a sense this was a variation on Fleming's ditch test, but was more accurate and provided a better method of quantifying the strength of penicillin being tested. Florey had started something similar as part of his own research program and Heatley essentially brought Florey's method to perfection. The cup-plate assay started with the usual agar-coated Petri dish. Onto the agar were put four or five little cups, actually small ceramic open-ended cylinders. The different samples of penicillin to be tested were put into the cylinders in measured amounts and the rest of the agar was seeded with the bacteria, which were being used as test organisms. After an appropriate time in the incubator the plate would come out covered by the whitish or yellow growth of germs except for empty, or blank, disks around the little cups. The radius of the clear areas gave a measurement of the strength of the penicillin placed in the cups. One carefully preserved, but quite arbitrary, penicillin solution served as a standard. Thus was born the "Oxford unit" of penicillin. It never had any real meaning in an absolute sense, and nowadays we can only make educated guesses about how much penicillin, in our modern units of measurement, was really present in an Oxford unit. It must have been very little, because it is usually more convenient nowadays, both for dosing patients and for assessing manufacture, to count in millions of units (megaunits).

The making and measuring of penicillin were, therefore, well under way quite early in the Oxford story. Extracting and purifying the drug were the big problems.

Chain had discovered that the best way to start the extraction was by making the crude penicillin-containing medium rather acid and then mixing with ether, which took up the penicillin and left the first large block of impurities behind in the medium. But the only way to stop the penicillin being entirely destroyed by the acidification at this stage was to keep it very cool, at around 0° C. Using this method on a larger scale, as Heatley was trying to do, involved the use of the refrigerated room which was part of the department's facilities. But since the ether and the medium had to be shaken together to achieve mixing, this meant that someone had to work inside the refrigerated room shaking large, gallon-sized glass bottles. So not only the penicillin but the operator also, was cooled to 0° C. Mufflers, gloves, overcoats, boots and woolen helmets were the dress-of-the-day for Heatley and any assistants he could get. His chief assistants were soon the "penicillin girls," who were recruited specially to help him and who made history, not only by manufacturing the first penicillin to be used to cure people but also by being the first women ever to be trusted to provide technical help within the portals of the Sir William Dunn School of Pathology of Oxford University. The first two were Ruth Callow, who was the sister of Chain's personal assistant, and Claire Inayat Khan; both had had some training in nursing. Later members of the penicillin girls were Betty Cooke, Peggy Gardner, Megan Lankester and Pat McKegney.

At first they shook the bottles of medium and ether violently to produce a good mix; but this also produced a nasty foaming emulsion, the problem that had troubled Ridley and Craddock years before and was to trouble the industrial manufacturers in the years to come. So they went to a method of gentle rolling of the bottles, which helped in overcoming production difficulties but doubtless was not so effective in keeping human circulations going in the refrigerated room. The bottles were the ones that had originally been designed for soft-drink concentrates.

At the same time Heatley was working to develop an automatic extraction plant, if plant it can be called. It was here that the Bodleian bookshelf came into the picture. The bookshelves were a large free-standing unit made of stout oak. In the final model three of the large bottles were mounted upside down at the top of the shelves. One contained crude medium, the next contained ether and the third acid. In principle what happened was that the medium and the acid were fed into ice-cooled tubes to produce the cooled, acidified mixture desired. This mixture was fed into the top of a large spiral glass tube, technically known as a worm. The ether was fed into the bottom of the worm and forced upward inside the worm by the pressure of the gravity feed from the bottle at the top of the shelving. Thus a counter-current flow was set up, with the penicillin-containing acidified medium flowing down through the upward-going ether. Penicillin was extracted from the medium into the ether in this process and the penicillin-rich ether was collected at the top through a u-tube siphon, while the unwanted medium drained away at the bottom. The whole apparatus was fitted with a home-made system of electric relays which were activated whenever the level of liquid in one of the three feed bottles fell below a pre-set mark, and the relays rang electric bells to warn the operator that fresh supplies were needed.

In the very early stages of production, at the time for the first mouse experiments, the ether was allowed to evaporate off after it, and the penicillin it contained, had been mixed with water. The remainder was freeze-dried to produce the penicillin powder with which the first experiments were made. Then Heatley had the idea that the penicillin might be back-extracted from the ether into another solvent, neutral amyl acetate. This idea, which might seem fairly obvious now, considering that penicillin was known to be more active nearer neutral pH, only occurred after "much creaking of the brain" (Heatley's words). At first Chain thought it would not work, but was quite willing to let it be tried, to demonstrate his point of view. In fact it did work, and then they took the whole idea even further and used amyl acetate as the main solvent instead of ether, and it continued to work. Amyl acetate had a number of extra advantages which soon showed up; it was less inflammable for one thing, and less of it was lost in the extraction process to go down the drain with the unwanted medium after the penicillin had been extracted. In fact, it was much better as long as people could stand the smell which was like that of nail varnish. Another minor improvement was the use of phosphoric acid in the initial acidification.

The automatic extraction apparatus reached its final form in January 1941, and Heatley was able to claim that production had increased a thousandfold in 1940. But the apparatus dealt with only twelve liters of fluid an hour, and with that they had to be satisfied throughout 1941.

In the meantime, the mouse experiments had been successful enough to lead Florey to demand extra production of the mold fluid as early as May 1940 and a significant advance had also been made, in response to that demand. Heatley had seen that growing the mold in the standard conical glass flasks of the laboratory was a terrible waste of space and stacking room in the incubators and in the autoclave used for sterilizing the flasks. What was needed was a vessel which provided a larger surface area of liquid medium on which the mold could grow, and a depth of medium of only about one and a half centimeters; and which would stack one on top of the other. He tried milk bottles on their sides, pie dishes, square biscuit-tins, and even bedpans, and worked in this way for many weeks. Eventually he decided that only a specially designed vessel would do the job. Taking into account the size of his shelves in incubator and autoclave, he decided he wanted more or less oblong vessels, only two and a half inches deep and with main dimensions ten and a half by eight and a half inches. They should be rough on the outside for good stacking and to prevent slipping, and smooth on the inside to make for easy cleaning and sterilizing. Finally they must have a spout at one end, sticking upward slightly. This spout was needed to allow the operation of the pistol-like device which was used for extracting the penicillin-containing medium and replacing it with air until fresh medium could be put under the mold. But a few inquiries showed that it would be quite impossible to obtain such vessels made in glass under the conditions of wartime England. Delivery from factories suffering from bombing and filled with priority government orders would be at least six months, and the mold for such a vessel would cost £500 to make.

It was typical of Florey's expert leadership that it was at this stage of impasse that he helped in solving the problem. He had a friend, a general practitioner, who worked in Stoke-on-Trent, the "capital" of the Potteries area, where most of the country's chinaware and ceramics factories are concentrated. He sent this doctor sketches of what was required and asked him to find out if there was any firm that would be willing to make such objects. The doctor soon achieved success with the firm of James McIntyre and Company which had a factory in Burslem, and he sent a telegram to Florey informing him of the chance to have his vessels made. Heatley set off next day, but the journey from Oxford up through the industrial Midlands was slow, as air-raids disrupted the train service. It was not until the following morning, October 31, that he could reach the pottery.

But the potters had not been hanging about waiting for him to turn up. When he arrived three prototype vessels had been roughed out in clay, and the modeler produced a final version with his knife as Heatley told him exactly what was wanted. Three trial vessels, fired and glazed, that arrived in Oxford on November 18, were found to be thoroughly satisfactory. The main batch of 174 vessels was ready on December 23 as promised. Heatley was ready for the vessels, too. He had borrowed a van, obtaining gasoline (the records do not describe precisely how this was done) and had arrived at McIntyre's pottery on the evening of December 22 in cold, but clear, weather. His queries about loading the 174 vessels were answered by "We'll see to that" and when Heatley got back from his hotel, first thing on the following morning, he found that the job had been done. He drove back to Oxford and spent the rest of the day with his assistant, Mr. George Glister, unpacking the van, washing the vessels, filling them with medium and sterilizing them in the autoclave. Christmas Day 1940, was spent inoculating the vessels with mold spores.

In parallel with the production work of Heatley and his colleagues, the penicillin girls, the chemists led by Chain and Abraham were toiling away equally heroically. In a sense they were working on two different levels. They had to invent techniques to purify the penicillin from the mold juice to such an extent that it could be used for biological experiments and the early treatment of patients. At the level of academic "pure" chemistry—the level at which these men were normally accustomed to working—their effort was aimed at producing really "pure" penicillin, penicillin completely without contaminants so that the antibiotic could be studied in detail and its molecular structure worked out. No chemist would be satisfied with a substance that simply cured; they had to know exactly how it was constructed, which atoms of which sort were placed where in the molecule. Only with a full knowledge could they seriously propose better methods of production, or how the drug acted to cure people, or, eventually, how to synthesize penicillin so that production would no longer depend on the unreliable behavior of the living molds.

Their technological solutions have already been described. At the level of pure chemistry the instability of penicillin presented even more severe problems. At first they tried to overcome this instability by creating salts of penicillin; that is, they tried to get it to combine with metals to produce crystals in the same sort of way chemists produce crystals of substances like copper sulphate. They tried adding to the brownish penicillin liquid copper, zinc, cadmium, mercury, lead, nickel, even uranium, the metal which at that very time was a subject of such interest to an entirely different and secret set of scientific investigations. But all these metals simply destroyed the activity of the penicillin. Then they tried organic bases: quinine, cinchonine, acridine, proflavine. All useless. Then ketones and alcohols. Still no success.

Chemical methods—techniques depending on causing chemical reactions in which the penicillin would bind with some other substances so that it could be extracted—having failed, they turned to physical methods. This was where they started chromatography with their concentrated penicillin juice diluted with water. No luck. Then, at Abraham's suggestion, they went back to the stage where the penicillin had been in solution with ether and tried pouring this down the packed tube. This time something happened: four clearly different colored bands appeared in the alumina powder where different substances in the original mixture had adhered to the alumina powder at different distances down the tube. When the powder was carefully spooned out of the tube with spatulas it became clear that the topmost brown band contained very little penicillin. Eighty percent of the penicillin, judged by its activity, was concentrated in the second band, which had a pale yellowish color. The dark brown band and the purplish band near the bottom of the tube contained only impurities.

So by taking only the yellowish powder from the second band (with the uncolored powder just above and below it to allow for inaccuracies and to save as much of the penicillin as possible) and repeatedly washing it in a buffer solution, all the penicillin could be flushed off the alumina powder and huge proportions of impurities were left behind in the packed glass tube.

This was the stage they had reached when penicillin as a drug was first tried on a human, the fatally-ill cancer patient who immediately developed fever and rigor, revealing that the penicillin being produced in quantity by Heatley still contained toxic impurities. And so the chemists were immediately able to apply chromatography to the "clinical" drug and purify it enough for Florey and Fletcher to go on with their successful human experiments. But the chemists had to pursue the antibiotic at their own deeper level.

At this stage they were preparing the mold juice that Heatley produced by the following techniques. First they cooled the mold juice to just above freezing point and acidified it with phosphoric acid. This mixture was added to amyl acetate and the penicillin passed into solution in the amyl acetate. To every two liters of amyl acetate they then added one liter of water, shook the mixture thoroughly and added alkali to reduce the acidity. The penicillin then migrated to the water and, when allowed to settle, the mixture separated into two clear layers of water and amyl acetate. Not only were impurities left behind in the amyl acetate but the penicillin had been concentrated into a solution of just one liter from the original two. The penicillin-containing water was then mixed with another two liters of the original penicillin-containing amyl acetate. Again penicillin migrated from amyl acetate to water and further concentration and purification had been achieved. This process was repeated ten times so that a twentyfold concentration of penicillin was achieved.

Filtration by passing the water and penicillin through a bed of bone charcoal was the next stage. Then the penicillin had to be persuaded to go into solution with ether so that the chromatography could be carried out. The watery solution was cooled to 40° F and acidified once again and mixed with one third of a liter of ether. Three times this operation was done till all the penicillin in one liter of water had passed into one liter of ether. Then the chromatography could be performed.

The band of yellow-stained alumina powder containing the penicillin then went into a seven-and-a-half-hour process of washing four times in a buffer solution, that is, a solution neutral between acid and alkali. This left the penicillin dissolved in six liters of solution. This was cooled and acidified again (because the penicillin would only accept acidification if it was cooled) and mixed with two liters of ether. The process was repeated three times with fresh supplies of ether each time. Then the mixture was neutralized again with alkali and added to one fifth the quantity of water. This reconcentrated the penicillin and left the yellowish pigment behind in the ether.

Next another purification by chromatography was deemed necessary. So the whole process of cooling, acidification and back into solution with the ether was begun again. Down the tube (a smaller one this time), wash with buffer, recover from buffer with ether, and pass back into water once again. And now they could, by adding barium and evaporating the water, at long last get the barium salt of penicillin in crystal form. It was actually a yellowish powder, and the yellowish color told its own tale of pigment and impurities being still present.

The only thing to do was the same thing all over again. Dissolve the barium salt of penicillin in water and extract the penicillin into amyl acetate. Eventually Chain and Abraham carried out three further stages of chromatography in addition to the ones we have already followed through. This gave them something like 500 units of penicillin per milligram of the final powder, where they had started with perhaps half a unit of active penicillin per milligram. They still had to use freeze-drying for the final evaporation of the barium salt of penicillin.

This technique was only applied to the pure chemistry processes, and was not at this stage being used for production of the early drug for clinical tests. Yet the myth of penicillin usually insists that it was only the freeze-drying technique that made penicillin possible.

All this work took Chain and Abraham well into 1941. And although they did not know it then they still had penicillin that was, strictly speaking, half impure. It was not till 1945 that crystals of pure penicillin would be made and analyzed by x-ray diffraction techniques to settle the formula and structure of the molecule once and for all. By then penicillin had been taken to the U.S.A. and the final solution of the chemical definition of penicillin came as much from American as British chemists.

The final purification plant was built in the Animal Post-Mortem House of the Sir William Dunn School of Pathology. This extraordinary building had been bequeathed to the scientists of the 1940s by an earlier generation who had plainly prepared for the possibility that post-mortems on rhinoceroses or elephants might one day be of value to the study of pathology. In 1942 Dr. A. Gordon Sanders and James Kent converted it into the world's first factory for producing penicillin, though its output was still pathetically small and not really enough even for full-scale clinical trials of penicillin. The process used was still essentially the same as that constructed on the basis of the Bodleian library's bookshelves, but there were variations such as the deliberate emulsifying of the mixture of mold juice and amyl acetate and their subsequent separation with a centrifuge. There was also the introduction of an extra purification cycle using chloroform instead of amyl acetate. The final plant included a number of items rarely found in a modern chemical-engineering factory: there was an ordinary domestic bath, a milk cooler, many milk churns, and a bronze letterbox. Some of the pumping was achieved by pumps which had started life circulating water in an aquarium. Nevertheless, this plant could process 160 liters of the mold juice in a three-hour run. Then it had to stop so that a gummy substance could be cleaned by hand from the bowl of the centrifuge. The small quantities of rich mahogany-colored fluid that the plant produced had to be run through the chromatograph by hand in a final preparation for clinical or experimental use.

I have used the rather dramatic word heroic to describe the days of 1940, 1941 and 1942 in the Sir William Dunn School of Pathology at Oxford. For a start these were wartime days, days when the Battle of Britain was being fought in the air a hundred miles to the south and east, days and nights when British towns and cities were being bombed. Oxford was fortunate to escape heavy bombing raids despite the presence of many automobile factories on the outskirts. But the scientists involved in the work had to spend some of their time queuing for rationed food. They welcomed many of their turns of firewatching duty, for these enabled them to work on in their laboratories at night. The baths and milk churns and library shelves were used because nothing else could be ordered or manufactured or bought.

But this was the first time a university department had ever found itself in such a situation. No one else had ever before discovered a naturally occurring life-saving drug, still less a drug that could save lives from so many different infections. Quite apart from the wartime emergency conditions there was none of today's administrative machinery that can be brought into play to help an important discovery along from the laboratory to the factory.

Florey and his men were pioneering. Pioneering firstly in the intellectual field by showing that there could be such a thing as chemotherapy, that there could be a naturally occurring drug which would cure many different infectious diseases. They were pioneering also in chemical engineering, in chemical laboratory techniques and in clinical medicine, for they had to work out just how and in what quantities their new drug should be applied to suffering patients.

It was against this dramatic background that Florey made

the biggest decision of his career. He decided that pioneering was not good enough in itself. He decided that wartime England was not the right place to develop his wonderful discovery, whatever it might mean to him and his colleagues. He decided he must seek help from America.

Chapter 12
PRODUCING PENICILLIN

FLOREY HAS LEFT no account of how he came to make his great decision. There is no record of any ministry or government agency asking him to go. He seems to have discussed the matter only with Sir Edward Mellanby, the secretary of the Medical Research Council. And he arranged the financing of the journey privately, with Dr. Warren Weaver of the Rockefeller Foundation, the man who dealt with his original application for money to investigate those "bacterial antagonists" which included penicillin.

Florey gave the impression to those who interviewed him that he had decided on his own account that the government was too busy with the war to spare the time, the finance or the material to launch a drive to manufacture the drug on the basis of only a few clinical experiments; six cases only in the spring of 1941. But certainly he had made his decision to go to America by April 1941, only three months after his first unsuccessful attempt to cure the Oxford policeman with penicillin. His objective in going to America was not, at first, the starting of really large-scale production. Heatley writes:

> Laboratory production could not be increased much more and, once he had good clinical evidence to present, Florey went to America (which was then not at war) under the auspices of the Rockefeller Foundation, with the object of trying to interest the Americans and persuade one or more commercial firms to prepare enough penicillin to treat a further score or more cases, which would have enabled its clinical value to be rigorously assessed. Without such additional proof it could hardly be expected that any firm would undertake large-scale production. It seems that Florey had approached the Rockefeller Foundation by the middle of April, if not earlier, and, the necessary formalities having been completed in secrecy . . .

What Heatley does not note is that some time in these crucial first three months of 1941 Florey realized the military value of penicillin. It is only at this stage that the mention of penicillin for treating war wounds first appears.

The Medical Research Council had, at all times, supported some of the work in Florey's department, although its claim to have supported the penicillin work right from the start seems dubious. The secretary, Sir Edward Mellanby, had been largely responsible for Florey's appointment at Oxford and was throughout these years Florey's principal support and mentor in official circles. Early in 1941 Florey received information through a private letter that the Germans, acting through Swiss contacts, were anxious to examine penicillin. He sent the letter off to Mellanby because he was concerned from the military point of view, writing: "I enclose this letter for you to see and it seems very undesirable to me that the Swiss should be allowed access to penicillin and that, through them it should go to the Germans. I think it would be well worthwhile to issue instructions to the National Type Collection Laboratories telling them not to issue sample cultures of *Penicillium notatum* to anyone with possible enemy connection.

You might also think it worthwhile sending a note to Fleming or anyone else who might have the mould, although I do not know anyone else myself."

Mellanby wrote back reassuringly that it was nothing to worry about, adding, "After all, you are so far ahead it seems that no one else can compete with you."

But soon afterward Mellanby wrote again to Florey, who had obviously consulted with him yet again. "Dear Florey: After discussing this with you, I have come to the conclusion that the only way that this most important matter [of penicillin production] may be pursued is for you and Heatley to go to the United States of America for three months.

"This is a subject of the highest medical importance and it is quite clear that you cannot get this substance made by firms in this country. I regard it as most important that you go to America and get the facilities there under way."

It is known for certain that Florey had approached several of the major chemical and pharmaceutical companies in England for help, and had received what amounted to "the brush-off." But Florey never admitted precisely which companies he approached. Undoubtedly some of the pharmaceutical companies followed up the *Lancet* paper of August 1940—"Penicillin as a chemotherapeutic agent"—and made inquiries at the Oxford laboratories putting some of their research staff to work on the new field. Masters quotes Florey as saying that he definitely approached "a chemical firm" which went so far as to say that they "would do their best" to produce some penicillin for him. But they produced nothing.

The memoirs of the scientists may, however, be unfair to these British firms. Imperial Chemical Industries Ltd. were able to produce small amounts of penicillin for Florey's clinical tests by as early as the first months of 1942, and by September of 1942 Burroughs Wellcome were ordering very large numbers of milk churns in order to produce penicillin on a fairly large scale. Of course management, staff and factories of the chemical and pharmaceutical companies were fully stretched at the time under wartime pressures. Probably even more important was the specter, or prospect, of synthesizing the new drug. This was where the sulphonamides, Ehrlich's antisyphilitic (Salvarsan), and even the comparatively recently discovered vitamins laid a false trail in the minds of scientists and industrialists alike, for all were either synthetic materials or had been analyzed and successfully synthesized. They offered examples of chemicals which could be manufactured from comparatively cheap and simple basic materials and were therefore susceptible to economical and carefully controlled factory production. Penicillin manufacture at this stage depended on highly unreliable and variable growth by living organisms followed by a complicated purification stage which was nowhere near a fully developed industrial process capable of being efficiently controlled. Any company that sank thousands of pounds on setting up a plant to perform these rather primitive operations was in danger of finding that they had lost all their money before they even started production, if the chemists were to discover the structure of penicillin and a simple way to synthesize it. We can hardly condemn those who thought that Chain and Abraham were close to success in total purification by 1941, or who could not foresee that penicillin would not be synthesized economically right up to the present day.

Yet from Florey's point of view—the scientists' point of view—larger production than they could achieve in their laboratories and animal houses was essential at this stage to provide material for proper clinical trials on human patients, for more intensive work on the pure chemistry, and even for the development of better production methods themselves. In June 1941, Florey and Heatley set out in a blacked-out airplane, via an unknown airport, to Lisbon, the brightly lit capital of neutral Portugal. They arrived there on June 28 with freeze-dried strains of Fleming's mold in test-tubes in their baggage. Three days of relaxation in what seemed to Heatley a "non-rationed paradise" were somewhat marred by worry about what the heat was doing to the precious contents of the test-tubes. The wartime Clipper flight took them via the

Azores and Bermuda and landed them in New York on July 3. Still worried about the effects of heat on the mold, they faced Independence Day with every office and laboratory closed. So Florey, on that first day, could only manage a visit to the Rockefeller Foundation to tell Dr. Alan Gregg of the results he had so far obtained with penicillin. Heatley remembers this important presentation as being "quiet and factual."

On Independence Day Florey went to visit Dr. and Mrs. John F. Fulton at New Haven, Connecticut. The Fultons were old friends and had given hospitality and shelter to Florey's children when they were evacuated from England at the beginning of the war. As soon as the holiday was over Dr. Fulton took Florey to see his friend Dr. Ross Harrison, chairman of the National Research Council. Harrison suggested that the man most likely to help was Dr. Charles Thom, the mycologist, the very man who had, at Raistrick's request ten years before, identified Fleming's strain of the mold as *Penicillin notatum.* Thom saw Florey in Washington on July 9 and took him directly to see Dr. Percy A. Wells of the U.S. Department of Agriculture. From this meeting came the suggestion that the Department of Agriculture's Northern Regional Research Laboratory at Peoria, Illinois, would be the best place to pursue penicillin's development because of the very large fermentation division which had just been built there.

Wells in fact sent a telegram to Peoria warning them to have a cabinet of fermentation trays ready for Florey when he arrived. And on July 14 Florey and Heatley arrived at Peoria, where the essential research, which finally enabled penicillin to go into production, would shortly be done.

Peoria itself was something new to the two British scientists. It was still in the building stage at the time they arrived, though the fermentation division itself was completed. It had facilities on a scale then undreamed-of in Britain. And, in the broadest sense, it was part of the Roosevelt New Deal program. The department's field of work was in applying research to the agricultural products of the Midwest and the Northwest, which in practice meant corn. A corresponding Federal

Laboratory under the Department of Agriculture had been set up in the South which equally dealt mostly with research on cotton. The Director of Peoria was Dr. E. Orville May and the head of the fermentation division was Dr. Robert D. Coghill. They immediately promised full cooperation when Florey and Heatley arrived and Coghill mentioned the possibility of "deep fermentation" in his first conversation with Florey. Florey was to remember this later when deep fermentation proved to be the answer to the economical and large-scale production of penicillin. Coghill was apparently equally impressed by Florey. His memory of that first meeting was: "They sold us the problem."

But the very first problem faced at Peoria was to get the freeze-dried specimens of Fleming's mold to grow. They had spent just over two weeks in test-tubes in the British scientists' baggage, being dragged around through the summer heat of Lisbon, New York and Washington. Heatley remembers "it was at first feared they might have died out at the high temperatures encountered since leaving England." Slowly and with difficulty they were persuaded to germinate again and fresh cultures were founded in Peoria's magnificent facilities. Then Dr. Andrew J. Moyer, a biochemist on the Peoria staff, was set to work with Heatley. Heatley was to stay in the U.S. laboratory for six months handing on the techniques that had been developed at Oxford, including such dull but scientifically vital procedures such as the method for assaying the activity of penicillin.

There was no fresh yeast available at Peoria at that time. Fresh yeast was, it will be remembered, a valuable addition to the synthetic Czapek-Dox medium which increased the yield of penicillin produced by the mold into the culture fluid. Moyer suggested the use of corn-steep liquor instead of yeast as an addition to the medium, and immediately it proved not only to work but to be better than yeast at inducing the mold to increase its output of penicillin. Corn-steep liquor is a by-product of the process of extracting starch from corn. It is notorious within the industry for providing a home and a nutritious substrate for unwanted bacteria and molds. Work on corn-steep liquor—how it could be discouraged from welcoming contaminants, how it might eventually be used in some practical way instead of being just an unwanted by-product—was just the sort of problem that Peoria had been set up to solve. But from Moyer's valuable discovery much trouble was to spring. For, when viewed from the British side of the Atlantic, A.J. Moyer stands out as one of the chief villains of the story.

Moyer and Heatley were working jointly on the penicillin project. Heatley was being paid by the Rockefeller Foundation, as part of the arrangement under which he and Florey had traveled to America. Moyer, of course, was on the Peoria staff, and there was an agreement between Rockefeller and Peoria, in the usual terms, that any results of their work should be published jointly and any royalties should be shared between the foundation and Peoria.

Heatley spent a few days away from the laboratory and when he returned he found that Moyer had pushed up the yield of penicillin from the mold even further. Many additional nutrients were being tried out in a fairly comprehensive program and eventually lactose was found to be another very useful component of the medium. But when Heatley started assaying Moyer's new output he found him curiously cagey about what had been added in addition to the corn-steep liquor. Nevertheless, they wrote up a joint paper on their work. Moyer showed Heatley a final draft shortly before the Englishman prepared to return to Oxford. He accepted a few last-minute minor amendments from the Englishman, who then left. After the war it was discovered by Heatley that Moyer had published the paper in his own name only. It was on the basis of this paper that Moyer filed three patents on methods of production of penicillin. The essence of these patents is the use of corn-steep liquor and lactose in the medium for growing penicillin molds. These are Patents 13674, 13675 and 13676, filed in the Patent Office of Great Britain, the first important patents to mention the word penicillin. They were to be followed by many other patents covering the manufacture of the first antibiotic, patents filed by both British and U.S. companies, most of which are now useless.

The story that Florey "gave away" the British patent right on penicillin to the U.S.A., the myth that American industry made millions of dollars from the patenting and sales of what was essentially an invention by British scientists, is based on these patents of Moyer's. The myth is completely untrue. The irony is that Moyer never made a penny out of these patents. As an employee of Peoria the ruling was that any patents made out of penicillin research should be equally shared between Peoria and the Rockefeller Foundation who were financing the work. The ruling did not cover employees filing patents in foreign countries, however, and Moyer appears to have acted within his rights in claiming the British patents. Nevertheless, his seniors were most annoyed when it was disclosed that he had filed these patents, and, under pressure by Coghill, the U.S. government departments involved, notably the Department of Agriculture, made sure by unofficial methods that he received no payments against these patent rights.

Later in this work Moyer discovered that the addition of phenylacetic acid to the medium persuaded the mold to produce much more penicillin of the type that had a benzyl side-chain. This was penicillin G, benzylpenicillin, for many years the penicillin of choice for clinical use. Moyer made considerable sums of money from this discovery. And Moyer remains a curiously enigmatic character. Despite what happened, Heatley retains memories of a man who was personally very kind and helpful to him. Yet he was "the most violently anti-British man I have ever come across, Pennsylvania-Dutch in origins and renowned for stubbornness."

In fact, the first use of penicillin to cure a patient systemically, that is, by the injection of the drug so that it acted against bacteria within the bodily system, had been achieved in America long before Florey and Heatley arrived, even before the Oxford policeman had been treated. The original paper by the Oxford team, published in the *Lancet,* had arrived in America in August 1940. Within five weeks Dr. Martin Henry Dawson, of Columbia University, was treating a patient at the Presbyterian Hospital in New York with penicillin injections. His small team consisted of Karl Meyer, working on the chemical extraction of the penicillin, and Dr. Gladys Hobby doing the microbiology. The mold strain they used came from Dr. Roger Reid, that other American pioneer of penicillin who had failed in the same way as Raistrick and Fleming himself in the mid-1930s. Dr. Dawson conducted a sort of personal crusade against the rather rare but usually fatal condition of bacterial endocarditis, and the first patient ever to be given penicillin by injection was a sufferer from this disease, Aaron Alston. The treatment was not a success, the patient died and Dr. Dawson concluded: "The drug preparations were extremely crude and, moreover, extremely low in potency." Dawson wrote to Chain in Oxford and asked for specimens of his penicillium mold, hoping it would produce more penicillin. The cultures were immediately sent off from Oxford, but on arrival in the United States they never produced any penicillin at all. Relying, therefore, entirely on Dr. Roger Reid's culture Dawson's team started a process of manufacture remarkably similar to the Oxford work, with stacks of hundreds of bottles in the classrooms of Columbia University. Karl Meyer did brilliant work in producing penicillin for further clinical cases, and he is, in the opinion of some American experts, the most under-rated figure in the history of penicillin.

Nevertheless, insufficient supplies of the drug meant that Dawson could not record startlingly successful results in the four further cases of bacterial endocarditis that he treated. He got better results with cases of staphylococcal infection. In May 1941, Dawson, Hobby and Meyer reported to a meeting of the American Society for Clinical Investigation. In a handwritten summary to his paper Dawson concluded that "it would appear that penicillin is a chemotherapeutic agent of great potential significance."

Dawson, by this time, was becoming aware of his increasing symptoms of myasthenia gravis, a condition in which the muscles slowly lose all their power. He continued to work until his death in 1945 but his disease steadily reduced his productivity. Although he stands out as the first in America to recognize and use penicillin he necessarily slips out of the main story.

The campaign to persuade America, and especially American industry, of the importance of producing penicillin in some quantity was left to Florey. Florey visited eight of the greatest chemical and pharmaceutical manufacturers in the North American continent: Lilly, Merck, Sharpe and Dohme, Lederle, Squibb, Pfizer, Eastman in the U.S.A. and Connaught Laboratories in Canada. "Several of these companies showed interest, but the only effective steps towards production at that stage came first from Merck and Co. Inc., and then from E.R. Squibb and Sons and Chas. Pfizer and Co. Inc.," according to Professor Stewart. But the initial nature of the difficulties Florey faced in approaching industry is best described by Professor Hare. By a series of coincidences which illustrate how small is the world of progressive medicine at any one time, Professor Hare was then working at the Connaught Laboratories in Toronto. Connaught was officially attached to the University in Toronto, but was in fact a vast commercial production laboratory. Largely the creation of one man, Dr. J.G. Fitzgerald, Connaught manufactured vaccines to finance its own medical research; on a huge New World scale it did what the old Inoculation Department of St. Mary's had also done. Hare, who had been offered a post there in 1936, describes Florey's visit with remarkable frankness and humility:

> In August 1941 I was suddenly called to the office of Dr. R.D. Defries who had become the Director of the Connaught Laboratories following the death of Dr. Fitzgerald. He introduced me to Professor Howard Florey and Dr. N.G. Heatley, who he informed me had been studying a substance called penicillin of which I might possibly have heard. Florey then told the almost incredible story of how . . . they had succeeded in producing mould juice in porcelain containers; and how Chain had purified sufficient for the treatment of six moribund patients with staphylococcal infections, only two of whom had died and then only because they had run out of penicillin.

It then emerged that the main purpose of their visit was to persuade us to make penicillin in quantity. . . . But when we ascertained exactly what this meant the problem became formidable. Large rooms would be required merely to act as incubators in which to grow the mould. And the method of purification used at that time seemed difficult to adapt for large-scale production. [With a copy of Florey's paper] in our hands we consulted the chemists. When they asked us how we proposed to produce penicillin and we told them by the growth of mould in containers of some kind, they laughed at us and predicted that by the time we had spent a great deal of time, money, and energy on something so futile, they, the chemists, would have found a way to synthesise it. . . . We accordingly told Florey that we could not undertake the assignment. He was, naturally, disappointed and I do not think he ever forgave us. But he was, in fact, asking a great deal at that particular stage of the penicillin story. One of the most important requirements was the evolution of a method for large-scale production. . . . The second requirement was proof of the value of penicillin. When Florey came to see us it had only been used for staphylococcal infections. No one knew how it would behave when faced with other organisms under other conditions. I, for one, had not forgotten how dangerous it is to extrapolate in science, to assume that an agent that will cure infection by one species of microbe will behave in the same way when called upon to deal with other species. The arsenicals had taught me that lesson.

But on August 7, 1941, Florey made what turned out to be his breakthrough in the U.S.A. He went to see Dr. A.N. Richards, professor of pharmacology at the University of Pennsylvania in Philadelphia. Dr. Richards had just been appointed chairman of the Committee on Medical Research at the Office of Scientific Research and Development, but equally important he was also the man with whom Florey had worked fifteen years before when he had come to America on a Rockefeller Fellowship. Florey found that Richards promised "to see that everything possible was done to expedite the production of penicillin." And Richards was as good as his word.

Florey went back to Oxford in September 1941, but with Richards's backing, on October 2 the U.S. Committee on

Medical Research agreed to give priority to the production of penicillin. Incidentally, Dr. Vannevar Bush was in the chair at this meeting in his capacity as director of the Office of Scientific Research and Development. Six days later he called a meeting between government representatives and four of the big pharmaceutical firms. Merck at least emerged from this meeting having agreed to join a government-sponsored project on the research and production of penicillin. By October 20 the first technical conference on penicillin was held, with reports from Merck, from Dr. Thom and from the latest research at Peoria. At this meeting it was decided to speed up the tempo and a grant of a further $8000 was promised by the Committee on Medical Research. At the next technical meeting, on December 17, it was agreed that all research results from both government (i.e. Peoria) laboratories and from the commercial firms (mainly Merck at this stage) should be pooled through the Committee on Medical Research. Much had been achieved since Florey arrived in New York in the beginning of July, and all really on the basis of six clinical cases in distant Oxford.

But it was in this same month, December 1941, that the attack on Pearl Harbor took place. America was plunged into war and the penicillin which Florey had hoped for in order to extend his clinical studies never left the shores of America. Nevertheless, production of penicillin had been started on both sides of the Atlantic.

PRODUCTION IN THE UNITED STATES

The basis of all production of penicillin was the development research carried out at Peoria.

First there was the work by Moyer and Heatley improving the yield of the Fleming strain of mold by adding corn liquor and lactose to the medium. Whereas in Oxford Heatley had been producing about two units of penicillin (measured by the standard of his own Oxford unit of activity) in each milliliter of medium, his work with Moyer increased the yield to forty units of penicillin per milliliter of medium.

But at the same time Dr. Kenneth B. Raper, the mycologist at Peoria, began a world-wide search for other strains of penicillium mold capable of producing penicillin. In his own collection of molds he found a close relative of Fleming's strain, called NRRL 1249 B2 (NRRL standing for Northern Regional Research Laboratory, the proper name of Peoria), which produced more penicillin than Fleming's strain. He obtained the assistance of the U.S. Army Transport Command, and, from every corner of the globe, soil samples were sent to Raper's laboratory. From these samples he isolated many different organisms, each capable of producing penicillin in some quantity or other. (So much for the uniqueness of the spore that floated through Fleming's window from the dusty streets of Paddington in the mythical version of the penicillin story.)

But oddly enough it was on his own doorstep, practically, that Raper found the winner. One of his assistants, who soon earned herself the sad nickname of "Moldy Mary," was commissioned to go regularly into the market at Peoria and collect every type of mold she could find on waste fruit or on anything else. One day she came back with a rotten cantaloupe melon, and from this was isolated the strain NRRL 1951 B25, which became, in the course of time, the origin of most of the penicillin produced in the world. NRRL 1951 B25 was not actually a *Penicillium notatum*, a relative of Fleming's strain; it was a *Penicillium chrysogenum* and its particular advantage was that it would readily grow in a submerged state in deep fermentation. Also, this remarkable mold had a yield of penicillin far higher than anything found before.

By this time Dr. Robert D. Coghill, head of the fermentation division at Peoria, had built up a team of scientific workers every bit as efficient as the Oxford team, but doing entirely different types of work. The research at Peoria was essentially devoted to developing methods of producing penicillin more efficiently by bringing enormous resources to bear onto the problem. The hundreds of specimens of penicillium molds that Dr. Kenneth Raper collected were grown by his assistant, Mrs. Dorothy Alexander, and assayed for production of penicillin by W.H. Schmidt, working ten hours a day, seven days a week. Coghill's deputy as head of the division, Dr. George E. Ward, contributed himself to the technology of deep fermentation, while Drs. Frank H. Stodola and J.L. Wachtel worked on new methods of recovering penicillin from the brew more efficiently.

Meanwhile Coghill was coordinating a series of projects at Stanford University, the University of Wisconsin, the University of Minnesota and the Carnegie Institute at Cold Spring Harbor, N.Y. In Coghill's words:

> The objective was to obtain better penicillin-producing strains of the mould either by isolation from nature or by the production of mutations from previously known organisms by means of light, x-ray or chemicals. Among tens of thousands of mutants examined, a number of high yielding strains were thus obtained, the best of these being an x-ray induced mutant of *Penicillium chrysogenum*, NRRL 1951 B25, which was produced by Dr. Demerec, of the Carnegie Institution. This organism, known as X.1612, is now very widely used by the penicillin industry and is producing what formerly would have been considered fantastic yields—as much as 500 units per millilitre in pilot plant equipment and consistent yields of over 300 units per millilitre in the large-sized fermenters of some industrial plants.

That is to say that with the proficiency of the new corn-steep liquor medium and the new man-made strain of mold, production was 250 times what Oxford had been getting, and all within a few months of Florey's trip to the U.S. (Later there was an even greater improvement in penicillin-producing powers when the University of Wisconsin workers produced a mutant by ultraviolet radiation which could yield 900 units of penicillin per milliliter of medium. This was called WIS. Q. 176.) The article in which Dr. Coghill wrote the above was the first to reveal to the public what had been done. It appeared in *Chemical and Engineering News* in 1945, and yet Coghill still had to write, a few paragraphs further along, "The chemistry of penicillin, as of this writing, is still classified as secret."

It must be remembered that penicillin had become, from 1941 on, a wartime project, a drug that would save the soldiers and airmen of one side from death and probably enable them to return to battle, while the Germans and Japanese, not possessing it, would be at a disadvantage. This strictly military view of penicillin was bound to be the prevailing one throughout the years when penicillin went into production.

The coming of war in December 1941 entirely changed the industrial prospects for penicillin in North America, as well as depriving Florey back in England of his promised supplies. The Squibb Company joined with Merck in a collaborative program and agreed to make information on penicillin production available to all other interested firms. They also agreed to hand over all the penicillin they made to the Committee on Medical Research, which would organize the distribution to approved doctors and hospitals for extensive clinical trials. The trials themselves had already been set into motion, administratively at least, by an earlier meeting in January 1942, when the National Research Council set up a committee under Dr. Perrin H. Long. It was decided to try the new drug first against the staphylococci, which was where Florey had had his first successes.

The Merck-Squibb agreement had been reached in February 1942. By March there was enough penicillin available for clinical testing to begin. This performance alone justifies Professor Stewart's remark: "The ready and incredibly rapid cooperation of these firms as well as the U.S. government were key factors in the production of penicillin for therapeutic purposes."

The first American patient to be treated with industrially manufactured penicillin was the wife of a Professor at Yale. In March 1942 she was on the point of death suffering from puerperal fever and widespread septicemia. She had failed to respond to treatment with sulphonamides. Penicillin produced by the Merck company was given intravenously, that is, dripped directly into a vein. And in the U.S.A., as in Britain in the previous year, the "miraculous" results of penicillin were seen. The patient recovered remarkably quickly.

But in the next three months the total production of penicillin in America was only enough for ten more cases to be treated with the antibiotic. The results were uniformly encouraging and slowly penicillin production began to go up. By the end of 1942 a further 200 cases had been treated and penicillin was beginning to be used against germs other than the blood-poisoning staphylococci and streptococci. It was tried out, for instance, against gonorrhea and a success rate of 100 percent was reported to the committee before the end of 1942.

This increasing number of reports of clinical success from highly respected medical institutions—such as the Mayo Clinic and Columbia University (where Dr. Dawson and Gladys Hobby continued their work)—steadily swayed the argument in favor of penicillin. The only failures seemed to be when penicillin was used in too small a dose. From Dr. Coghill's point of view the fundamental question was, "Is penicillin good enough to justify the great expense of overcoming the great production difficulties. If so how much will the armed forces need and how can we improve existing production methods?"

By 1943 it had been decided to go full ahead for penicillin production on a large scale. The War Production Board officially sponsored and supported the drive. Six big American companies were now involved: Merck and Squibb, of course, and Pfizer, Abbott, Winthrop and Commercial Solvents. And this was soon followed by an absolute penicillin boom. Everyone who could get into the business did so and there were soon at least eighteen more firms of various sizes and degrees of reputability also involved.

> One was so successful an adaptation of a plant for the production of mushroom spawn that, for a time, its owner was looked upon as the coming man in the industry. But some were started by amateurs who seemed to be doing it as much for fun as from patriotic or pecuniary motives. One was in a shop in the main street of a little country town with a basement full of inflammable liquids, and was the worst fire trap I have ever seen. Perhaps that is why the chemist in charge of it chewed gum the whole of the

three hours we were with him. But the most remarkable was run by a businessman employing a bacteriological technique entirely his own invention, based mostly on old whiskey bottles sterilised by steam direct from a boiler on the point of bursting, in the Stygian gloom of a derelict factory in the meaner part of Brooklyn and staffed entirely by negresses. Unorthodox some of them may have been, but the fact remains that the Americans got their penicillin.

American readers who may feel put off by the stuffiness of this British description of their activities should note the admiring justness of the last sentence. The description comes from Professor Hare who had by now been put in charge of the project for manufacturing penicillin at the Connaught Laboratories in Toronto, since the clinical successes of 1942 had caused the Canadians to regret their initial refusal of Florey's request.

And the Americans certainly did produce penicillin. In the first six months of 1943 the total U.S. production of penicillin was about 800 million units; but in the next six months just over 20 billion units were produced. Because of the very small strength of the first Oxford unit (see p.176), penicillin has to be given in what seems to be enormous doses. One million units is quite a normal quantity for a single injection of penicillin into an ordinary patient nowadays. In fact, one billion units is roughly able to deal with 1,000 serious cases of illness.

In the next year, 1944, U.S. production of penicillin was increased eightyfold to 1633 billion units. And in the following year it increased fourfold to some 6800 billion units. In 1945 the monthly production figures fell from July to October because, of all ironies, there was a shortage of adequate quality corn-steep liquor.

At the same time the price tumbled steadily. In 1943 the Office of Scientific Research and Development, the parent body of the Committee on Medical Research, offered a price of $200 per million units of penicillin. By 1945 the price had come down to six dollars for a million units.

Demand, however, increased as quickly as the price came

down, though probably this was not the traditional operation of the forces of the marketplace; it was more a case of people wanting to be cured of disease at any price. From July 1943, however, when production really got going, penicillin had been virtually rationed in the U.S. (The official wording is that the War Production Board had placed penicillin under allocation.) Military requirements took up as much as eighty-five percent of all production right up until 1945, when the military demands decreased to only about thirty percent of the very much increased output. But even then only 2700 recognized hospitals received supplies of penicillin for civilian use. The distribution of penicillin within the U.S. had a rather complicated history with the factors of the personal need of the patient clashing with the perfectly proper desire of the scientists to obtain as much information about the clinical value and uses of the drug as was possible. At first, Dr. Chester Keefer of the Committee on Medical Research had the difficult task of reconciling these conflicting claims, and he achieved what was widely respected as a thoroughly equitable dispensing of the rare material. By April 1944 the supply of penicillin was too great for Dr. Keefer to manage, but still too little for all the civilian needs. The Penicillin Producers Industry Advisory Committee then worked out a plan for distributing it through nominated hospitals. At first there were only 1000 hospitals on this list and the Civilian Penicillin Distribution Unit in Chicago had to clear all orders for penicillin. The number of depot hospitals holding supplies of penicillin increased by 1945 to 2700 and through the depots a further 5000 hospitals could get their supplies. By the end of 1945, penicillin was virtually freely available through the normal commercial channels in the U.S.A., and by then it was allowed to be exported freely. When export restrictions were finally lifted the unusual situation arose that export demands were equal to total internal consumption. By the end of 1945 the U.S.A. was exporting 200 billion units a month and consuming the same amount.

This total 1945 production was estimated at a value of sixty million dollars, despite the drop in the price of penicillin. Dr.

Coghill declares that this had been produced by a total investment of twenty-five million dollars in buildings and equipment over the previous three years. Rather less than one third of this capital had come from the U.S. government. Investment in penicillin production had plainly been well worthwhile. But it had been more worthwhile for some than for others. For while a small "surface culture" plant might have cost some $350,000 to bring into production, a big "deep fermentation" plant required an investment of as much as three million dollars.

The true secret of the enormous American production of penicillin, the reason the Americans within three years were able to satisfy their own wartime needs for penicillin and most of the rest of the world's needs, lay in the development of deep fermentation. This was the Americans' greatest single contribution to the history of penicillin. Likewise, it is their justification for rejecting the British "sour grapes" charge of having "stolen" the scientific discovery of penicillin. What the Americans did by discovering deep fermentation was to make the whole of the modern antibiotics industry a practical proposition. If the British, mainly at Oxford, discovered penicillin, the Americans found the way of making it available to the world.

Penicillin was first observed by Fleming after a mold had grown on the surface of the medium in one of his Petri dishes. In all the subsequent work the mold had been grown on the surface of the medium, producing its penicillin in the liquid underneath it. Following this line, all the early production of penicillin—at Oxford as much as in the U.S. industry—had been surface culture of the mold. The technical debate of the early days of the penicillin industry, and this applied in America as much as in Britain, was between "bottle-culture" and "tray-culture." In wartime Britain ordinary glass milk bottles laid on their sides were much used, though of course there were Heatley's specially designed ceramic culture vessels and later there were similarly shaped glass flasks. The advantage of closed bottles or flasks was that, once the medium had been seeded with spores of the mold on the surface, the neck could be closed with aseptic material and contaminating germs of other sorts could be kept out. The alternative was to use trays full of medium, stacked on top of one another. The much larger surface area of medium obtainable in a tray gave the mold more room to grow, and therefore increased the production of penicillin in the medium below. But with tray-culture the whole room in which the trays were incubated had to be kept sterile, and the loss, if contamination did occur, was likely to be much greater than with bottles or flasks. As far back as Raistrick's work, it had been shown that the penicillin production of the mold reached a maximum after a certain number of days (the exact timing depended on the nature of the medium and the temperature at which it was incubated). Afterward the production of penicillin fell off sharply. Production of penicillin was, therefore, essentially a batch-production industry, with loads of flasks or trays being planted out with spores and then left for a set period; after which the whole of the batch would be harvested and the chemical processing of the medium to recover and purify the penicillin would be started.

If a penicillium strain could be found which would grow and produce penicillin while submerged in the medium the whole process would be changed. For a start the entire production of penicillin by the mold would be increased by a whole dimension. Molds growing submerged in a soup of medium would have the whole volume of the container at their disposal instead of just the surface of the medium. Furthermore the costly, slow and labor-intensive task of seeding the mold spores into tens of thousands of bottles, flasks or trays would be eliminated.

Peoria had set itself the task of trying to make deep fermentation possible from Coghill's very first meeting with Florey. There were three main problems to be solved. First a high-yielding strain of mold that would grow while submerged in medium had to be found. This was achieved when NRRL 1951 B25 was isolated from the moldy cantaloupe melon. Then a way had to be found of supplying air that was completely sterile and free from contaminating organisms to the mold growing within the medium, for penicillium molds need air to grow. Furthermore, this air would have to be distributed throughout the container. Finally, the contents of the container would have to be stirred continuously so that the mold was continually furnished with fresh supplies of the nutrients contained in the medium, and again this would have to be done without introducing contaminants. In due course these problems became the chief task of the team assembled by Coghill at Peoria. But these problems were essentially problems of chemical engineering when it came to finding solutions on an industrial scale. It is at this point that the next important name enters the story of penicillin: Chas. Pfizer and Co.

It is the biggest single failing of the myth about penicillin that it ignores the technological breakthrough of deep fermentation, a breakthrough that was every bit as vital to the successful development of penicillin as any of the more dramatic laboratory work. An essential feature of this development was that Pfizer was not a pharmaceutical firm at all when it went into the penicillin manufacturing field. The company was, however, one of the pioneers of deep-fermentation technique in its normal course of business as a supplier of chemicals and ingredients to the food and drink industry. This detachment from the traditions of the pharmaceutical industry seems to have given Pfizer a freedom of thought and a fresh approach which enabled it to make some very bold decisions when it finally decided to go in for penicillin production. This freedom from the conventions of pharmaceutical thinking seems also to have been a trait of many of Pfizer's managers as individuals.

In the early days of struggling to make penicillin production a viable industrial enterprise one of the Pfizer directors, John L. Smith, a small, rather stiff-looking man, was approached by a Brooklyn physician in June 1943 who asked for some of the still rare penicillin to treat a young girl dying of infectious endocarditis. Smith protested that penicillin was under official allocation and in any case there was no reason to think it would be effective in a case of endocarditis. The doctor somehow persuaded him to come and see the girl in the hospital and Smith was so moved that he agreed to break the regulations and give some of the penicillin. After three days of direct intravenous drip treatment the girl was so much improved that thereafter the penicillin was given by injection and in a month she was cured completely. Smith had visited the hospital daily during the crucial period and was so impressed with what he saw that he continued to supply the doctor with penicillin until the doctor was using 200,000 units a day on a variety of cases including others suffering from endocarditis. The National Research Council insisted on the allocation regulations being observed since there was still no "convincing" evidence of penicillin being effective against endocarditis. Smith, however, was even more convinced by what he saw in the hospital than by the demands of the N.R.C., so he continued to break the regulations. More important, he conveyed his personal knowledge and enthusiasm for penicillin into the Pfizer organization. Nevertheless, the key figure in Pfizer's successful introduction of deep fermentation as *the* method of penicillin production was John McKeen.

In a sense, much depended on the history of the Pfizer company. In 1848 twenty-two-year-old Charles Pfizer, a chemist's apprentice, and his cousin, a trained confectioner, Charles Erhart, left their hometown of Ludwigsburg in the Kingdom of Württemburg and emigrated to America. This was at the time when the German chemical industry was beginning its rise to world dominance. Within a year of their arrival the two young men had formed a partnership, obtained the use of a small building in Brooklyn and set up business as chemical manufacturers specializing in chemicals that were not then manufactured in the U.S.A. Their first product was Santonin, a substance then widely used for getting rid of worms. In the Pfizer company's own mythology it is believed that Pfizer's chemical skill was very much complemented by his cousin's expertise in confectionery, because the product was sold in cones, rather like sweets and candies, and the presentation achieved by the new firm brought success.

Iodine, and its relatives in the antiseptic field, were the next area into which they ventured. But their real and lasting success came when they started the bulk manufacture of basic materials for the food and drink industries, using their European connections as a source of raw material. Shortly after the Civil War had caused a major change in the commercial relations between the U.S.A. and Europe, Pfizer started importing argols and refining them into tartaric acid and cream of tartar for the baking, confectionery, and soft-drinks industries. Previously tartaric acid had been imported from the wine-making areas of France and Germany. Then in 1880 Pfizer began importing crude citrus-juice concentrates from Italy and the Mediterranean countries and processing these into citric acid and its derivatives to serve other needs of the U.S. food and drink industry.

It was this line of business that led Pfizer into the fermentation business, for supplies of its raw material were threatened by the approach of World War I. A laboratory was set up in 1914 and after nine years' work a method was found of making citric acid through the fermentation of sugar; in other words, a micro-organism was discovered which, when fed on sugar, would convert the sugar into citric acid as a by-product of its own metabolism. (Penicillium molds of the right type produce penicillin when fed on a nutrient medium in just this way.) The Pfizer plant for producing citric acid by fermentation was opened in 1923. Four years later when Italy banned the export of citrate of lime Pfizer was left in a commanding position in the supply of this widely used material in the U.S.A.

Naturally the company followed up its first research success and soon found a fermentation process for the production of gluconic acid, a staple raw material not only in the food and drink industries but also in textiles and pharmaceuticals. By the end of the 1930s Pfizer was the world's first mass-producer of gluconic acid.

Fumaric acid, likewise widely used in the food industry as an acidifying agent, was the next thing that Pfizer tried to manufacture. In producing gluconic acid the company had used submerged organisms: the deep-fermentation technique. Pfizer tried the same technique for fumaric acid, and duly found a mold which would produce it. The company's main research effort just before the war was directed precisely at these problems but, whereas gluconic acid had been easy to produce, all the problems that were later to be met in penicillin production were found in trying to produce fumaric acid. There were problems of stirring the medium whilst retaining complete sterility; there were problems of keeping the medium at a precise neutrality; there were problems with foaming just as in penicillin.

In 1941 the last of the Pfizers active in the company (Emile Pfizer) died. John L. Smith, whom we have seen cheerfully breaking the penicillin allocation regulations, was primarily a chemist and had led the company's work in citric-acid fermentation. He became president of the company in 1944. The chief chemical engineer was John E. McKeen (who was to succeed Smith as president in 1949), and it was he who pushed Pfizer into being among the first three U.S. firms to produce any penicillin (Merck and Squibb were the other two). Pfizer started like the others with surface culture techniques. But McKeen was quickest to follow up the scientific work of the Peoria team into deep fermentation. By August 1943, Pfizer had built a pilot plant for deep fermentation of penicillin. And then came McKeen's big decision: to go straight up to large-scale production. From the chemical-engineering point of view some very courageous scaling-up was required here. And the company undoubtedly met some severe teething troubles. But this was just where the experience gained on fumaric-acid production paid off. It has been estimated that the fumaric-acid production experience saved Pfizer two years' trouble-shooting work at this stage.

By 1944 Pfizer's deep-fermentation penicillin plant was in action. By the end of the war this one company was making more than half the total world production of penicillin by using the new technique. Merck, which had its own pre-war experience of fermentation techniques, was following hard in the same direction, and Commercial Solvents was also deeply involved in deep-fermentation production.

So fast had the situation changed that Dr. Coghill, writing only in 1945, said, "This trend to the submerged process has been so marked that there is only one bottle plant operating in the United States today." Some of the deep-fermentation plants, he reported, were already using production units so big that the vat fermentors contained 12,000 gallons of nutrient medium.

But by 1945 there was also penicillin production in comparatively small bottle plants in Australia and Canada (where Professor Hare and his colleagues had eventually converted a training school for Presbyterian ministers into a penicillin factory), and a considerable industry in Britain producing enough of the drug to supply the country's own needs. But in Britain all production was by the surface method; deep-fermentation techniques were almost unknown to the chemical industry there. And in 1944 the leading British manufacturers gave up the struggle to remain independent and came to America to obtain licenses on the deep-fermentation techniques.

PRODUCTION IN BRITAIN

Contrary to the widespread belief inculcated by the penicillin myth, the British chemical industry (with much help from the admiralty) had successfully supplied all of Britain's wartime military needs for penicillin. But the story of the production of penicillin in Britain in the 1940s is very different from the dynamic drive of the foundation of the new industry that occurred in the U.S.A. It is a story of bombs and milk churns and gasoline rationing; a story that eventually ended in surrender, and the expensive purchase of licenses to manufacture by the superior American techniques.

Florey returned to England from America in autumn 1941, with a promise of supplies of penicillin to follow him. But by January 1942, he found that his team at Oxford and Imperial Chemical Industries had provided enough penicillin for him to start a reasonably large clinical trial of the new drug. (The fact that I.C.I. could produce penicillin as early as January 1942 effectively disproves the story that Florey went to America because *no* British firm would do anything about the new drug.)

The big trial of penicillin in the first months of 1942 was one of Florey's major contributions to the history of penicillin. It was this trial that established the value of penicillin on a firm scientific basis. Florey had only had six cases to talk about when he went to America and his paucity of results led in many cases (such as that reported by Professor Hare) to his meeting a frosty reception. Florey performed a major scientific feat in establishing the usefulness of penicillin in these few weeks of 1942 in wartime Britain. And his claim to priority in establishing the clinical value of penicillin is undisputed, for the Americans had not yet started making penicillin and could only carry out their very first test in March 1942.

Further, Florey established in this same series of trials the whole basis of the dosages of penicillin required for different cases. He showed how the effects of the antibiotic varied between different methods of administering the drug. He described how to measure the levels of penicillin in the bloodstream of the patient being treated. And he demonstrated how patients' differing clinical conditions affected the drug regime that should be prescribed. He did all this while treating just fifteen patients systemically, i.e., by introducing penicillin into the whole system through the bloodstream. One hundred and seventy-two other patients were treated with penicillin by local administration of the drug. Professor Stewart thirteen years later wrote admiringly of Florey's work at this time: "It shows what can be accomplished under conditions of shortage—of assistance, of money, of apparatus and (not least) of penicillin itself—by critical investigators."

One case among Florey's early cases was particularly important. It was a two-month-old child critically ill with infection of the bones at many different places (multiple foci of osteomyelitis). The successful results in this case gave the first indications of what penicillin dosage was actually required. And by a curious coincidence it was a similar case of the same disease that was among the first to establish the value of the first of the semi-synthetic penicillins exactly twenty years later.

Florey's work was followed by other trials in the same year, though still with minutely small supplies of the drug. Colebrook (who figures in this story very much earlier as a member of the staff of the Inoculation Department at St. Mary's Hospital, Paddington) did some of the tests in the Burns Unit at Glasgow Royal Infirmary. The first use of penicillin in treating war wounds was recorded at this time, again as part of the early test program. Dr. Dennis C. Bodenham at the Princess Mary Royal Air Force Hospital at Halton, for instance, helped to confirm work being done at the Burns Unit at Oxford. penicillin in combination with sulphanilamide would dispose of the cocci in wounds and thus prevent sepsis. A little penicillin was also spared for testing at the Scottish Military Hospital in Egypt, where Colonel Robert J.V. Pulvertaft achieved remarkable results using the antibiotic on wounded men from the desert army.

Busy and involved in his clinical trials as he was, Florey apparently took some time to realize that the promised supplies of penicillin from America were not going to reach him at all. He did not launch a determined campaign to get the government to support a major drive for the manufacture of penicillin till the middle of the year. He had, however, made a small step earlier than this, in fact as early as February 1942 (we shall return to this critically important step later). But in August 1942, he received surprisingly potent help from a most unexpected quarter. For at this stage Professor Alexander Fleming suddenly steps back right into the middle of the story.

It was on August 6, 1942, that Fleming telephoned to Florey and asked him whether he could have some penicillin for use on a patient. The patient was a fifty-two-year-old oculist, a friend of Fleming's. The man had become ill on June 18 running a continuous though not very high temperature. He was taken into St. Mary's Hospital on July 17 and his condition continued to baffle the doctors. It was rather like meningitis since his neck was stiff and he was drowsy, but his temperature remained only just over 100° F. A sample of the cerebrospinal fluid showed no trace of any causative organism. Treatment with one of the sulphonamides reduced his temperature somewhat, but at the end of a week's course of the drug his fever returned and his symptoms worsened with mental confusion and loss of control of his functions.

Further samples of cerebrospinal fluid produced no positive results for any known germ. By the end of July no progress had been made toward a diagnosis and the patient had developed a persistent hiccough which the doctors were unable to control. Fleming was personally very distressed by the state of his friend, and on August 1 another sample of cerebrospinal fluid was taken. Fleming, as bacteriologist, tried culturing this on a rather unusual medium: a very soft mixture of glucose and agar. And immediately he found a streptococcus. Further tests from yet another sample of fluid three days later proved that the streptococcus was indeed the organism causing the damage, because when mixed with a sample of the patient's blood it immediately caused agglutination (the clumping together of red blood cells which signifies that the patient has developed an immune reaction and manufactured antibodies against the organism). At this same time Fleming showed, by his old methods of culturing on agar plates and using the ditch test, that the sulpha drugs would not affect or kill this particular streptococcus. But his own crude penicillin, the simple mold juice which was still regularly prepared in his laboratory for nothing more than bacteriological tests, did kill the germ.

Fleming knew about Florey's work; he had read the Oxford papers in the *Lancet* with delight. He had even visited the Oxford team briefly and met both Florey and Chain. His request to Florey on August 6 for supplies of penicillin was, however, based on the scientific results of his own tests and not on any sentiment. He was justified in asking for penicillin when he had shown that mold juice would kill the streptococcus on his agar plates.

Florey had very little penicillin available, but it was the only penicillin in Britain at that moment. He agreed to Fleming's request on one condition only, that Fleming should allow him to include the case in the clinical trials of penicillin. Naturally Fleming agreed, and Florey caught the next train to Paddington carrying his entire supply of penicillin with him. He went directly to St. Mary's and showed Fleming the yellow powder, the first time Fleming had ever seen the substance. Florey told Fleming what he had discovered in recent months about the clinical use of penicillin and immediately returned to Oxford, promising to send further supplies as soon as they were available.

Fleming's case notes for the patient on August 6 read: "The patient was in a very bad state and appeared to be dying. He took little food; had been for days drowsy with occasional bouts of extreme restlessness; now drowsy, comatose, wandering and rambling; had been suffering from uncontrollable hiccoughs for ten days. On the evening of Aug 6th two-hourly muscular injections of penicillin were begun. In twenty-four hours the patient was mentally clearer, his hiccoughs had disappeared and head retraction was less marked. Temperature had fallen to 97° F."

But there the improvement remained and no further progress could be seen. Florey duly sent extra supplies of penicillin and the patient received sixty injections in five days. Still he was no better and other measures obviously had to be tried. Fleming decided to inject penicillin directly into the spinal theca so that it would get into the cerebrospinal fluid where the germ was known to be. This had never been done with penicillin but Fleming had always been known for his remarkably steady hand. He wisely rang Florey first for his advice but Florey could only say it had never been done.

Since the case was desperate Fleming went ahead and injected 5000 units of penicillin into the spinal theca. Later that day Florey rang back to say that he had just done the experiment of injecting penicillin into the spinal theca of a cat. The cat had died immediately. Fleming was able to say that his patient was still alive. And he went ahead and gave further spinal injections to the oculist in the following days, while continuing the regular intramuscular injections as well. Eventually the patient complained that he was suffering from lack of sleep since he was woken every two hours for an injection. So the night injections were stopped and on August 19 a final spinal injection of 5000 units of penicillin was given.

On August 28 the patient got up for the first time. On September 9 the hospital records show that he left, "apparently well." And well he remained for at least four years until he vanishes from history. Again the word "miraculous" crops up—this time from Fleming himself. Just over one and a half million units of penicillin (i.e., a fairly average dose) had saved a man from what seemed certain death and sent him away cured.

Fleming immediately set himself to influence the government to take up the manufacture of penicillin on a large scale. He went to Raistrick and the conversation was as follows:

> FLEMING: "What is the best way of getting the Government to take it up?"
> RAISTRICK: "The best way would be to go straight to the Prime Minister. Do you know Mr. Churchill?"
> FLEMING: "No. But I know the Minister of Supply."
> RAISTRICK: "I'd go to him straight away."

And that is exactly what Fleming did. The minister of supply, Sir Andrew Duncan, a fellow Scotsman, was indeed a friend of Fleming. A telephone call from Fleming was enough to fix a meeting, and Fleming impressed the minister with what he had just seen penicillin do for one of his patients. Sir Andrew Duncan called up Sir Cecil Weir, the director general of stores and equipment in his ministry, who had charge of the directorate of medical supplies, and ordered him to do everything in his power to get penicillin production moving.

The first big official meeting in Britain to discuss the large-scale production of penicillin took place, on Sir Andrew Duncan's instruction, on September 25, 1942, with Sir Cecil Weir in the chair. Raistrick would say for many years afterward that it would never have happened but for the fact that all three— Fleming, Duncan and Weir—were fellow Scots. The books (such as Masters's and Maurois's) leave it at that, with the clear implication that Fleming was largely responsible for bringing the government in and for starting the large-scale production of penicillin in Britain. But the evidence shows clearly that it was not so. Once again, it was not as simple as that.

The evidence also shows that I.C.I. was producing penicillin by the beginning of 1942—only in small quantities, it is true, but enough to help Florey to do his clinical tests. The Glaxo Company commissioned its first small penicillin-producing plant in a disused cheese factory at Aylesbury in Buckinghamshire in the first half of 1942. This factory had been set up with backing from the ministry of supply, as a direct scaling-up of the methods used in the Oxford laboratory. Within Glaxo the man who urged this move most strongly was Mr. (later Sir) Harry Jephcott and the man in charge of setting up the factory was Mr. Herbert W. Palmer. Mr. Palmer remembers first hearing about penicillin on a wartime train journey to the Colwyn Bay resort in North Wales. His traveling companion, an executive of Boots Pure Drug Co., tossed across to him a copy of Florey's 1941 *Lancet* paper.

Glaxo went on to set up two further penicillin factories, one at Watford, just to the north of London, in the top story of a building otherwise used as a rubber-vulcanizing plant, and the third in a converted cattle food factory at Stratford in East London. In all these activities they acted as direct agents for the ministry of supply. (Another large pharmaceutical company, Burroughs Wellcome, had also entered the manufacturing field in early 1942.)

Florey himself had made one of the most significant moves as far back as February 1942, when, through his friend and ally, the Oxford chemistry professor Sir Robert Robinson, he had approached the comparatively small chemical firm of Kemball, Bishop and Co., with the object, at first, of simply getting larger supplies of the initial mold juice. Sir Robert

Robinson had been consultant to Kemball, Bishop for some time, and had already provided help on the chemical side of Florey's work by making staff and facilities available at his own Dyson Perrins Organic Chemistry Department (which is in the same road, South Parks Road, Oxford, as the Sir William Dunn School of Pathology). Sir Robert was a man with considerable influence in British official circles and was later to be president of the Royal Society.

As a result of Sir Robert's negotiation the following letter was written on February 23, 1942, by Mr. John Edward Whitehall, managing director of Kemball, Bishop, to Professor Florey:

> We have heard today from Professor Sir Robert Robinson that you have consented to make us acquainted with the method for the production of penicillin and also to supply us with a specimen culture. Sir Robert suggests that we should send someone to Oxford to see the equipment and to bring away full details. We propose, with your permission, to send a Biologist and an Organic Chemist. The latter, Mr. J.G. Barnes, may be known to you as the possessor of an Oxford Blue for running [Ah yes, this was really England]. . . . We were approached by the Wellcome Foundation Ltd. [the research side of the Burroughs Wellcome pharmaceutical company] in respect of this matter some months ago when they informed us that the quantity they wanted was 10,000 gallons and quickly. This would have meant putting out of production other things of great national importance, and consequently we were not in a position to take further interest in the matter. But Sir Robert informs us that help on a small scale would be very welcome and with our experience in work of this kind we shall hope to make it a success with the aid of the valuable information which you so kindly and generously are willing to make known to us.

The two scientists from Kemball, Bishop, were at Oxford within the week, and Mr. John Gray Barnes (the athletics Blue) remembers that "as the group leader Florey gave us much of his time and went into great detail about the work they were doing." On March 2 Mr. Whitehall wrote again to Florey:

Mr. Barnes and Mr. Ward have brought back the cultures you kindly gave them and also the enlightenment on the production of penicillin. I therefore want to convey to you my Company's high appreciation of your kindness in supplying so freely the necessary information to enable us to begin our work and for the large amount of valuable personal time you placed at their disposal. I quite understand that the main object of this was not enlightenment for us but enlightenment to lead to production, which we shall most certainly try to accomplish.

But it was not going to be all that easy. On March 5 the Kemball, Bishop men tried to cultivate the strains of penicillium which Florey had given them (this was still Fleming's original strain). There was complete failure and after seven days they had to throw the test tubes away. Florey had to send them a second sample of the mold, which arrived on March 15. This time they did succeed in growing it.

Kemball, Bishop decided on the tray-culture method for growing large quantities of the mold. They selected two rooms in the basement of their factory at Bromley-by-Bow in East London. They installed air-filtration equipment to achieve sterility and air-cooling apparatus to get the temperature down to 24° C which is the optimum temperature for penicillium growth. The two rooms were equipped to take fifty trays each and each tray contained four gallons of medium, so the hope was to produce 400 gallons of penicillin-rich medium with each batch. The experimental work got off to a quick start; by March 25 the first tray was seeded and producing penicillin shortly thereafter. Kemball, Bishop, the small East London firm, can claim to be the first in the world to have produced penicillin on a scale larger than a glass bottle or a ceramic flask. Furthermore, the yield of penicillin in this first tray culture was seven units per milliliter of medium, considerably higher than anyone else had obtained at that time.

The engineering work did not go so quickly, which is hardly surprising since this part of London was still under fairly regular night bombing. Some idea of the conditions under which they worked can be gained from the story of the member of the night shift who entered the blacked-out works one evening and stumbled in the darkness over an obstruction in the road. The chief engineer took a torch to see what it was and found a 500-pound bomb embedded in the ground directly outside one of the windows with its detonator exposed and pointing upward. On another night the Germans were attacking with incendiary bombs. Several fell on the factory roof and the chief engineer had to deal with three of them while his colleague on firewatching duty, one of the workmen, dealt with two others.

"There's another fire," remarked the chief engineer as a building not far away started to blaze. "Yes and it's your house," responded the workman. He was quite right, too.

Luckily, the factory was never damaged by the bombing; much more serious problems were caused by contaminants which sometimes ruined an entire batch of penicillin cultures. It was not until the very end of August 1942, that Kemball, Bishop were ready to send Florey the first delivery of bulk penicillin-rich medium: precisely two milk churns full.

The ministry of supply was actively involved in obtaining at least some production of penicillin before any public pressure was applied to it. This is clear from the timing of the Glaxo factory building, and also from a reply by Sir Cecil Weir to Sir Andrew Duncan's first inquiries about penicillin production after his meeting with Fleming. Masters records that Weir replied to the Minister, "We've just been considering whether something could be done to get factory production going."

Certainly Florey had been in touch with the ministry before this, because in the first days of September he was negotiating to get a gasoline supply allocated for a weekly run by a lorry loaded with milk churns from Kemball, Bishop to his Oxford laboratories. Once Kemball, Bishop had started delivery the amount of penicillin medium available rapidly increased. It is clear from Florey's correspondence with Kemball, Bishop that two lots of two twelve-gallon milk churns had reached Oxford by train before September 22—indeed, one consignment had stood all night on Oxford station because the railway staff had failed to inform the laboratory of its arrival. It had not suffered. The letters about the lorry and the gas ration between Florey and Mr. Whitehall envisaged loads of twenty-five milk churns. And on September 28, just three days after the first historic meeting of the General Penicillin Committee, Florey wrote to Kemball, Bishop in these terms:

> As you will now know the Ministry of Supply is prepared to help in any way possible with the production of penicillin. As I have told you before, I consider your firm quite the most likely to be able to produce penicillin in quantity in the near future. Others have "plans," but translation of these "plans" into action is quite a different matter. I have the impression that now we have the backing of the Ministry of Supply and the Army as well, and they are not prepared to stand about and have the work held up for lack of material etc., we shall be all right. For the immediate future it can be said that if you apply to Mr. Denston of the Ministry of Supply for the milk churns to send us 200 gallons every ten days you will have no difficulty getting them. With regard to the petrol Mr. Denston will have to activate the Ministry of War Transport. Again I think they should have no difficulty getting it for you.

This is the letter of a man who had already done much pushing to get the production of penicillin going, and who had suffered considerable frustration at the hands of both government officials and industrialists. Nevertheless at this stage, September 1942, the fact remains that, judged by the number of clinical trials performed, the British pharmaceutical industry had produced marginally more penicillin than U.S. industry had yet turned out.

Florey had been invited to the first meeting of the General Penicillin Committee, which was held at Portland House in London on September 25, 1942 (this clearly shows that British officialdom was much slower than American to muster itself in support of penicillin). Florey had insisted that representatives of Kemball, Bishop be invited because they were "quite the most likely to be able to produce penicillin in appreciable quantities." There were six Ministry of Supply officials, two very senior officers from the Army Medical Directorate, Flem-

ing and Raistrick. Then there were men from I.C.I. and representatives from the Therapeutic Research Corporation (a
grouping of the main pharmaceutical firms of Britain, formed
under wartime pressure for pooling research work). They had
already agreed that work on penicillin research would be an
appropriate objective for their first major task. I.C.I., as we
have seen, had gone into penicillin production from the first.
The company was not a member of the T.R.C. and penicillin
was the very first venture of the British chemical giant into the
pharmaceutical field. I.C.I. had tried from the start to apply its
undoubted chemical-engineering expertise to what was for it
a new set of problems. The result was a slow start.

The meeting began auspiciously with Sir Cecil Weir, the
chairman, announcing that the Minister of Supply was "much
interested in the potentialities of penicillin" and had given
instructions that his department "should take steps to ensure
that all the available knowledge of this drug be pooled and
concentration and extension of production facilitated, even to
the extent of Government assistance, if required."

The industrial representatives assured the ministry that
there was full collaboration between the various firms in
T.R.C. and that collaboration between T.R.C. and I.C.I. was
well advanced. Most of the pharmaceutical firms had connections with American pharmaceutical interests, and there was
transatlantic exchange of information, as well as cross-linking
with university researchers. All seemed very smooth till Florey
spoke. The official minutes record:

> Professor Florey went on to say that, although American penicil-
> lin producers had been given free access some eighteen months
> ago to all the available information at the disposal of the School
> of Pathology, Oxford University, now, when the American pro-
> duction was on a moderate scale, it had not proved possible for
> him to obtain information from them as to their experiences, the
> Americans insisting that this information should be regarded as
> secret, and not to be imparted to anyone other than members of
> the T.R.C. and those working with it. He also referred to the
> patents which had been taken out by certain people. That state

of affairs was most unsatisfactory as Oxford University remained almost the largest penicillin producers in the country.

After this outburst it was rapidly agreed that T.R.C. would hand over the information it received from America "without restraint" to nominated independent research workers as well as Florey. Kemball, Bishop said that it, also, had American associates and would now have to see whether this barrier could be cleared in its case, too.

One obvious proposal—that all penicillin work should be concentrated in a new, large, high-powered research center— was rapidly rejected on the grounds that such a unit would be very vulnerable in wartime. For the same reason a proposal that industrial and production effort should be combined at one center was rejected. Various companies spoke of their plans for production on a larger scale, and the I.C.I. representative reported that his company was already producing 2000 liters a week of penicillin-containing medium.

The first arrangements were tentatively made for setting up a system for pooling and distributing all penicillin when it was produced. The meeting, ending with unanimous approval for controlling the public mentioning of penicillin in the scientific and lay press, produced results. Within two weeks Kemball, Bishop had got the milk churns they needed with ministry of supply assistance, and they had a gasoline allocation for their lorry. By October 13 the regular delivery of 150 gallons of crude penicillin liquor to Oxford had begun. Next the company started to try extracting penicillin from the liquor themselves, and two months later it was seeking ministry assistance to get the materials for an extraction and production plant.

But here one can see clearly that wartime shortages and the difficulties of applying purification techniques such as chromatography (the direct scaling-up of Florey's laboratory processes) held up the response of British industry, in contradistinction to the greater resources and bolder methods applied in America. It was September 1943, before Kemball, Bishop first started to produce penicillin, the drug, on an industrial scale from a rather makeshift plant. It was January 1944, before the plant was in full production, turning out twenty million units of penicillin a week, by which time U.S. national production was in the region of hundreds of billions of units a month.

The development of a number of small units using bottles and flasks for growing the mold by surface-culture techniques (in just such a way as Glaxo developed their penicillin production) was the response of the other British companies involved in penicillin production, companies such as Boots, Burroughs Wellcome and Distillers. From 1943 (the Sicily invasion campaign) the British pharmaceutical industry produced enough penicillin for the British military forces. But that production came essentially from rather makeshift plants whose principal feature to the outside observer's view was their conveyor systems, carrying glass flasks and bottles to the sterilizer, to the seeding department where large numbers of women injected mold spores into the flasks, to the incubator rooms, out of these rooms to the processing and extraction plant, and back to the sterilizer.

The interesting question is: Why were Kemball, Bishop the quickest in producing the crude liquor and why did Florey think they had the best chance of producing appreciable quantities of penicillin first? The answer must be that the firm was already a specialist in fermentation techniques. Not only was Kemball, Bishop almost exactly the British counterpart of Pfizer in America; it actually had agreements with Pfizer whereby the British firm obtained Pfizer know-how on the fermentation techniques for producing citric acid in exchange for Pfizer obtaining fourteen percent of the firm's shares. This agreement had been concluded in 1936, but none of Pfizer's know-how on submerged-culture techniques was included in the agreement. In 1959 Pfizer bought up the company completely.

The General Penicillin Committee concluded that they would have to promote a major British production drive for penicillin. At their meeting on July 8, 1943, it was agreed:

"There was general opinion that it would be a mistake for this country to rely on getting penicillin in any quantity from the U.S. before the end of 1944 and that the product was of such vital importance for the war effort that this country must take urgent steps to meet its own needs. Recent reports from the War Office indicated the value of penicillin in the treatment of war conditions."

And later, and perhaps in the long run a more significant statement: "Mr. Jephcott stated it was the intention of T.R.C. to extend production. . . . Using non-mechanical means a speedy increase in output could be obtained if sufficient labour (largely non-skilled) were available. Mechanization of production would retard output. Mr. Warburton [from the directorate of medical supplies in the Ministry of Supply] made it clear that urgency to increase supplies was the first consideration and the Ministry of Supply would give the utmost assistance to this end."

And so the British pharmaceutical industry never really considered, never perhaps had a chance of considering, any method of production except a scaled-up version of what Florey and Heatley, Chain and Abraham, had done in the laboratory.

This particular July meeting of the General Penicillin Committee dealt again with publicity and found it had run into a difficulty. It had succeeded in getting publication controlled and now found that its own workers could not publish their scientific results for each other's information. Rather pettishly it complained about inequality of treatment of scientific workers in the U.S.A. who were allowed to publish their results.

Of more importance are those Reports from the War Office indicating the "value of penicillin in the treatment of war conditions." The man behind these reports was Florey himself. He was not present at the Committee's July meeting for the very good reason that he was in North Africa personally supervising the first major applications of penicillin to war wounds. This was Florey's other great contribution to the history of penicillin, and its importance must never be underrated.

What Florey did in North Africa, working in the hospitals serving the Anglo-American invasion forces, was nothing less than to force a generation of practicing medical men to accept a medical revolution, to accept the antibiotic revolution, to accept that chemotherapy had arrived.

Florey's faith in the powers of penicillin was scientifically based on the results he himself had achieved in his clinical trials in 1942. But it is difficult to convince men that "a miracle" has happened and the reaction of doctors in the 1940s when they first saw penicillin at work on a patient was that it was "miraculous."

The technique—devised by Florey and those in British military hospitals and burns units who were collaborating in penicillin trials in 1942—of treating war wounds was, in layman's terms, to put penicillin and sulfa drugs into an open wound and then to sew up the wound. This was the exact opposite of all previous medical wisdom, which knew by harsh experience that to sew up a dirty wound containing earth or dust, scraps of clothing or other debris, was to invite fatal sepsis or gas gangrene. Florey personally supervised the military surgeons performing his methods of wound treatment. He even heard a visiting surgeon, peering over his shoulder at what was going on, mutter, "It's murder." The results, of course, proved Florey right. But it was very largely by his own force of character, backed by the earlier results he had achieved, that he brought penicillin into the medical armory as the most powerful drug then known, and all in a few months' work.

By 1944 British penicillin production was reaching a satisfactory figure, satisfactory at least for the wartime needs of the armed services. But it was all coming from the series of comparatively small bottle-and-tray plants which the various companies had set up in whatever buildings they could find. The question of post-war needs of penicillin for the civilian population then began to emerge, since it was quite clear that penicillin had come to stay. Various estimates of the likely national needs were put before the General Penicillin Committee.

Professor Raistrick was by now in charge of the national scheme for penicillin production and under his guidance preparations were made for the building of two large modern factories to put penicillin production on a satisfactory long-term basis. Sites were chosen at Speke (near Liverpool) and at Barnard Castle in County Durham. The Distillers Company was to build and run the Speke plant and Glaxo the Barnard Castle plant. Serious design studies were under way by the middle of 1944. By that time, too, the new and improved strains of penicillin-producing molds discovered at Peoria had been sent to Britain and the flow of scientific information between research teams on both sides of the Atlantic had been brought to a satisfactory level.

It was under these circumstances that news of the successful development of the deep-fermentation process reached Britain. Harry Jephcott of Glaxo and Dr. William R. Boon of I.C.I. were immediately dispatched to America by the ministry of supply. Before the end of 1944 the ministry of supply had been firmly told by the two companies that the future of penicillin production lay in the deep-fermentation plants. The ministry's reaction was slow, according to Mr. H.W. Palmer of Glaxo. After all, the building of the Barnard Castle plant had already begun.

Results from America provided more and more impressive evidence of the superiority of the submerged-culture methods and the ministry began to waver in the early months of 1945. Provision was then made in the plans of the new plants for stages that would allow for deep-fermentation techniques. This was enough for Jephcott. Before any decisions had been taken at the official level he signed agreements with Merck and Squibb for the purchase of their deep-fermentation technology. The other companies in the T.R.C., still working through the ministry of supply, regarded this as rather fast footwork, but by the summer of 1945 Glaxo had sent Palmer and three other men to Merck to learn enough of the techniques of stirring the enormous fermenter vats, of bubbling sterile air through them, and of the special devices used to inject mold spores into the vats, to enable them to supervise the building of deep-fermentation plants in Britain.

All further building at Barnard Castle was devoted to deep-fermentation production, and the Speke plant was built from the start for the new technique. Distillers Company had even obtained ministry of supply support for their own license agreement to buy the know-how from Commercial Solvents in America. By 1946 the new plants were coming on stream and the other companies were closing down their bottle plants and showing a tendency to bow out of the race, with the notable exceptions at that stage of Boots and I.C.I. The other companies asked, however, that they should share in a national scheme for the distribution of penicillin manufactured by the new plants. The General Penicillin Committee continued in existence long after the war to sort out problems like this.

In the harsh economic conditions and the dollar shortage that faced Britain after the end of the war, the decision to remain in the penicillin-production business and to continue to pay the license monies on the deep-fermentation technology was quite deliberate. Import of manufactured penicillin from America was forbidden on the grounds of dollar shortage.

The licenses that Glaxo, Distillers and others bought in 1945 ran for fifteen years. There is no doubt that British companies did pay many millions of pounds in license royalties over the years. It is a fascinating twist to the penicillin story, however, that before the license period was completed, the transatlantic balance of payments began to swing the other way as British companies established a world-wide patent hold on the semi-synthetic penicillins. Meanwhile, it is essential to point out that the license fees charged by the Americans on their deep-fermentation know-how were not merely reasonable, they were by ordinary commercial standards "modest." That is the official description by Glaxo. Furthermore, when world penicillin prices started to come down steeply in the late 1940s these license fees were reduced, not merely voluntarily reduced, but actually scaled down at the instigation of the U.S.

companies, notably by Merck. So much for the myth of the Americans racking penicillin profits out of the British discoverers of the drug.

Moreover, the American license agreements made no limitation upon British sales rights in any part of the world except America and Canada. In a meeting between the pharmaceutical industry and the ministry of supply on February 6, 1946, to discuss the peacetime distribution of penicillin once the new plants were in full production, the chairman, again Sir Cecil Weir, is minuted as saying: "Whilst it might be desirable to have a uniform selling price for the United Kingdom, so far as export was concerned it was essential to sell at the lowest possible price so as not to enter the export field at a disadvantage with the United States. It would be necessary to decide on the proportion for export, and whether it should be restricted to the lowest cost variety." The meeting then discussed whether the price per million units of penicillin should be fixed at five shillings or six shillings *above* the cost of production from the deep-fermentation plants so as to keep the bottle-type manufacture viable to enable a sufficiently low export price to be achieved.

So by 1946 penicillin was not only fully in production, it had become an element in the world-wide battle for sales and exports.

Chapter 13
PATENTS AND PUBLICITY

THE FIRST that the public knew of penicillin was on August 27, 1942, when the London *Times* carried an editorial, a leader, on the subject. There had been the two articles—both strictly scientific—reporting the work at Oxford, in the *Lancet* in 1940 and 1941. Then in the summer of 1942 the *Lancet* had published an editorial on penicillin, couched in cautious and rather professional medical language, urging the government to take more active steps to help industry produce penicillin. It was this policy that the *Times* leader supported.

Entitled "Penicillium," the article refers briefly to the observation of the fact that "a mould, *Penicillium notatum*, possessed strong antibacterial powers," giving no names or places, merely saying that it had happened "some thirteen years ago." Again naming no names, but stating that the work had been done in Oxford, the newspaper described the great power of the drug, its lack of toxicity and its advantages in attacking many germs not sensitive to the sulphonamides. After writing about "the alluring prospect," the *Times* ends by supporting the plea of the *Lancet* that "in view of the potentialities, methods for producing penicillin on a larger scale should be developed as quickly as possible."

This first public revelation of penicillin and its powers coincided exactly with Fleming's first successful treatment of a patient by penicillin therapy. This was the case of the oculist, who left the hospital on September 9, 1942. Fleming did not go to visit the minister of supply, Sir Andrew Duncan, until after his patient was cured, according to his biographer Maurois. It follows, therefore, that Fleming's intervention may not have been as important in stimulating the start of production as many writers have claimed. The evidence of dates makes it clear that the campaign to pressurize the government into action had already built up steam before Fleming spoke.

But the article in the *Times* was the signal for the action that started the myth of penicillin. The action took the form of a letter that appeared in the correspondence columns of the *Times* of August 31, 1942, under the title "Penicillin." The letter read:

> Sir, In the leading article on penicillin in your issue yesterday you refrained from putting the laurel wreath for this discovery round anybody's brow. I would, with your permission, supplement your article by pointing out that, on the principle *palmam qui meruit ferat* [roughly translated, "Give credit where credit's due"] it should be decreed to Professor Alexander Fleming at this research laboratory. For he is the discoverer of penicillin and was the author also of the original suggestion that this substance might prove to have important applications in medicine.

The letter was signed "Almroth E. Wright, Inoculation Department, St. Mary's Hospital, Paddington, W.2."

It was a fine act of loyalty to his colleague and supporter by "The Old Man." All the finer since the triumph of penicillin was the final blow to his own doctrines that "drugs are a delusion" and "stimulate the phagocytes."

But it was probably not entirely disinterested. Hospitals in those days in Britain depended almost entirely on voluntary contributions and the fees of private patients. Competition among hospitals for public acclaim, and competition among doctors for the fame or the connections that would bring them a large practice, was acute. To be known as the place where penicillin was discovered would not only be a feather in the cap of St. Mary's, but was also likely to be of considerable financial value. In 1942 a Health Service with hospitals financed from taxation was unthought of, except by socialist intellectuals, and was anathema to almost every doctor. This state of affairs will be more readily appreciated by a present-day American than by any inhabitant of Britain, where we have had a National Health Service for more than twenty years.

Whatever the mixture of motives behind Wright's letter—his last and perhaps his most lasting piece of public polemic—he thus started the myth of penicillin by placing the laurel wreath firmly on one man's brow. The first attempt to set matters right appeared on the first day after Wright's historic letter. It was another letter to the *Times* that appeared on September 1, 1942, written by Sir Robert Robinson, professor of organic chemistry, at the Dyson Perrins Laboratory at Oxford University. It read:

> Sir, Now that Sir Almroth Wright has so rightly drawn attention to the fact that penicillin was discovered by Professor Fleming, and has crowned him with a laurel wreath, a bouquet at least, and a handsome one, should be presented to Professor H.W. Florey, of the School of Pathology at this University. Toxic substances are produced by the mould alongside penicillin and Florey was the first to separate "therapeutic penicillin" and to demonstrate its value clinically. He and his team of collaborators, assisted by the Medical Research Council, have shown that penicillin is a practical proposition.

Sir Robert Robinson's letter was already powerless to stop the myth. Perhaps it was not strong enough in its terms to do so. That seems to have been the opinion of one of the few men who knew the truth at that time. Mr. J.E. Whitehall, managing director of Kemball, Bishop, who was at that time Florey's only industrial collaborator, wrote to Florey on September 1—a letter which has already been described for other historic reasons—that he agreed to provide the first industrial lot of penicillin to be made in Britain: two twelve-gallon milk churns of raw "mould juice." The letter ends with the following significant paragraph: "I was immensely pleased this morning to see in the current issue of the *Times* a letter from Sir Robert Robinson wherein he places matters connected with penicillin in their right perspective. I think that had I been writing, I should have been a little more explicit, but I can understand Sir Robert's desire not to hurt Professor Fleming."

The true balance of credit, then, was perfectly well known among the professionals involved in the business. But apparently none of them felt inclined to speak out more openly than Sir Robert Robinson had done for at least the next twenty-five years. Perhaps they felt they could not make themselves heard against the roars of applause that hailed Fleming. Florey never made any public attempt to redress the balance, and it was thirty years before Professor Chain made any public statement to this effect.

Within the scientific profession these three men, Fleming, Florey and Chain, have received due honor for their work. All three were elected Fellows of the Royal Society in London, the highest tribute of respect which British science has to offer. All three shared a Nobel prize, though at first the Nobel committee considered giving the prize to Fleming alone. All three were created Knights eventually, and Florey ended his life as Lord Florey, the president of the Royal Society. But the three men were split apart by their individual characters and their reactions to success.

When the first Oxford paper on "Penicillin as a chemotherapeutic agent" appeared in the *Lancet* in 1940, Fleming went up to Oxford to see "his" penicillin. Florey received him politely and showed him around the laboratories. Chain has admitted to his surprise at discovering who the visitor was: "I had never heard of Fleming except through reading his papers in my literature search. I frankly had assumed he was dead." Throughout the visit Fleming hardly said a word, and though this may have been his normal standard of uncommunicativeness, Chain was left with the impression that he had understood very little of what he was shown and that he had not the largeness of spirit to admit it. But it was the reaction to publicity that separated Fleming from Florey.

As soon as the news of penicillin reached the public and the two letters were published in the *Times* naming the men responsible, the storm of publicity broke. Professor Abraham's *Memoir of Lord Florey* relates what happened from the Oxford point of view:

> Fleming wrote to Florey on 2 September to say he was glad to see Robinson's letter [i.e., the letter to the *Times* from Sir Robert Robinson putting forward Florey's claims to the laurels]. He added "You are very lucky in Oxford to be out of range of reporters," but this was not in fact the case. The press sent representatives who received no welcome and little satisfaction from their visit and Florey stated in a letter to Sir Henry Dale that he had taken a firm line. He appears to have had two reasons for this, both commendable in themselves: an inherent dislike of publicity with its distracting effect on research; and the belief that it would lead to a demand for penicillin from members of the public which he could not then satisfy. One result, however, was that the press went where it was not rebuffed and published accounts of penicillin which were tendentious and one-sided, although the facts were mostly on record in the scientific literature.

Florey's biographer records the same facts more graphically: "It was a shock to Florey when the news corps arrived at the front door of the Sir William Dunn School. He immediately escaped through the back with instructions to his secretary, Mrs. Turner, to 'send them packing. I won't talk to them now. Tell them to come back next Thursday and I may give them ten minutes.'" And the comment follows: "A deep abhorrence of the media stayed with Florey for the rest of his life."

So the extraordinary situation arose that Fleming, notorious as a poor communicator, collected the first plaudits of the world through the press. Not unnaturally the Oxford team tended to blame him for the more bizarre stories that were printed. They did not know of his detached attitude of almost perverse amusement as he collected cuttings for "the Fleming myth." On the other hand Florey, well known in academic circles as a tough bargainer when it came to fighting for research funds, allowed the credit (which he could justly have claimed for himself and his team) to slip away through his disdainful treatment of the media. The Oxford team can hardly grumble because the press did not print stories that were not made available to them.

Florey's attitude to the press can be seen again in his leading the argument on the General Penicillin Committee for banning all publicity. And on that occasion, too, his antipathy to reporting of anything about penicillin in popular media led to unnecessary difficulties. (See Chapter 12.)

In defense of Florey's attitude, however, it must be said that he had already been made aware of some of the problems that publicity about penicillin might bring. In his first days as professor at Oxford he had earned the sobriquet of "bush-ranger of research" from another academic on account of his pursuit of grants for research work. When the Oxford team published their first paper ("Penicillin as a chemotherapeutic agent") in 1940 they gave pride of place in their acknowledgments of support to the Rockefeller Foundation. This spurred Sir Edward Mellanby to an immediate, though private, protest that the Medical Research Council had been unfairly given only a minor role in support of the work. Mellanby argued that the M.R.C. had provided grants totaling £1200 to various members of the team. He charged Florey with "wrong tactics . . . partly because if you have a good thing in your own country you might as well give it the proper credit and not follow those people who, in cases of research, find it more convenient to give foreigners boosts than their own colleagues. And having said that I salute you."

Florey's reply pointed out that the Rockefeller grant had given £1200 for the year in addition to £300 for Heatley, and he argued that the M.R.C. had provided only about £800 to support the penicillin work. Therefore he felt that the Rockefeller Foundation should be given the greater credit. The argument was not ill-tempered and Mellanby ended his later letter on the subject: "If you can get penicillin to cure cases of human bacterial infection I will forgive you a good deal more than your misdeeds in the present instance."

The question of the amount of support given to penicillin research became a matter of public debate in 1945 after Dr. Raymond B. Fosdick (president of the Rockefeller Foundation) mentioned in the foundation's Annual Report for 1944 not only the $5000 grant of 1939 and 1940, but also referred to a grant made to Florey as far back as 1936. This grant was for $1280 for "chemical work" and was not part of the history of penicillin, but Dr. Fosdick commented, "seldom has so small a contribution led to such momentous results." This was picked up by the London paper the *Evening News* which pointed out that if the American claim was true, then the Americans had every moral right to exploit the discovery which had depended on financial support from their country while the British government had been starving its native research. Mellanby again leapt into action, this time more publicly, declaring that the American claim (that a grant of £320 in 1936 had led to penicillin) was "grotesque." But a question in the House of Commons followed and the M.R.C. declared it had supported Florey to the tune of £7000 between 1927 and 1939.

At the root of this 1945 public controversy lay the question of the patents on penicillin. There had been no fumbling here, though the penicillin myth would tell you otherwise. There had been a very clear decision in Oxford in 1942 that it was unethical for a scientist to try to patent the outcome of pure research work, especially where this outcome was a substance of enormous medical potential. Chain, with his background knowledge of the German chemical industry and of the wider world outside the British university system, had battled furiously against this point of view.

Professor Abraham's *Memoir of Lord Florey* describes the situation as it was seen at the time:

> A different problem, which arose when it seemed that penicillin might be widely used in medicine, concerned the possibility of obtaining patent protection for the work done in the Sir William Dunn School of Pathology. Chain had strongly advocated patenting. At a meeting in 1942 Florey stated that the Oxford workers were not concerned with monetary reward, but were anxious to find a body such as the Medical Research Council willing to accept assignments and to undertake financial responsibility. It was probably then already too late for highly rewarding patents to have been obtained. But in any event no mechanism existed whereby patents could be handled by the University of Oxford or the Medical Research Council. Edward Mellanby, then Secretary of the Council, held strong views of principle that all such medical discoveries should be free. Officers of the Rockefeller Foundation felt that the possibility of a University obtaining money through royalties might put undesirable pressures on those in academic research. Thus nothing was done, for reasons which might have been admirable in a world with different economics, but seem almost irrelevant in the society in which we live. After the War, the climate of opinion changed.

Professor Chain confirms Abraham's statement of the forces and factors involved in the decision, but remembers that the actual discussions were nothing like so calm as the official *Memoir* implies. The arguments, especially between Chain and Mellanby, were in fact bitter and there is no doubt that Mellanby must take responsibility for the decision, right or wrong, not to attempt to patent.

A further important reason also existed making it impossible to patent penicillin in Britain. This was the simple fact that a drug, as such, could not be patented under British law at that time. The situation was only changed by the Patents Act of 1949, by which time it was realized that this was indeed "a world with different economics." Before 1942 no one had conceived the possibility that people could find or invent a "drug" which would be worth patenting.

Nevertheless, the question of patents on penicillin and the processes of its manufacture had been raised as early as the very first meeting of the General Penicillin Committee in September 1942 (see Chapter 12). It was Florey who had complained at that meeting that "certain people" had taken out patents covering aspects of penicillin. Both British and American companies filed for patents during the war years, and the matter continued to take up the time of the meetings of the General Penicillin Committee in Britain. It was eventually referred to higher levels on both sides of the Atlantic. The committee minutes for July 1943 show considerable agitation over the attempts by the U.S. company Winthrop Products Inc. and its associates to register the word penicillin or its Spanish equivalent throughout Central and South America as a trademark. T.R.C. and I.C.I. made formal legal opposition and there were diplomatic exchanges through the British mission in Washington. "Mr. Warburton stated that the U.S. government had found it difficult to bring pressure to bear. Winthrop Products Inc. had said their action was taken with the highest motives to prevent possible registration by parties who would monopolise the word as a trademark. They said they would make the name available to all firms in the U.S. and in this country." The meeting rather pompously "Agreed: That as Professor Fleming had given the name Penicillin to the product in 1929 as an open scientific name, every effort should be made to maintain this name as an open name." The matter was still coming up in the minutes in October.

But the real trouble began in 1945. On May 15 two Americans, J.W. Foster and L.E. McDaniel, filed patents at the British Patent Office for growing penicillin on corn-steep liquor. Sixteen days later Dr. A.J. Moyer had his applications filed for patents 13674, 13675 and 13676. The first was for culturing penicillin in eight different ways including submerged culture. The second mentioned thirty-nine different media for growing penicillin including several containing corn-steep liquor. The

third involved methods of regular addition of certain substances to the medium and the practice of withdrawing the
medium from under the mold and substituting fresh medium,
remarkably akin to Heatley's Oxford methods.

Moyer, as has been said before, made no money out of
these patents, but by 1945 censorship had been lifted, and the
Rockefeller Foundation report of Dr. Fosdick was being discussed. It was also, coincidentally, exactly the time at which the
British pharmaceutical industry, followed by the British government, realized that the bottle method of penicillin production had been defeated by deep fermentation. The bitter reali-
zation came home that Britain would have to take out licenses
and buy American technology on this method of producing
the drug.

It was from this coincidence of timing, rather than from the
facts, that the myth of penicillin patents has sprung. But the
only penicillin patents that were worth any real money before
1950 were those patents covering the chemical-engineering
details of the deep-fermentation process for producing not
only penicillin but also other antibiotics. These patents were
almost exclusively in the hands of four American companies,
Pfizer, Squibb, Merck and Commercial Solvents. And of these
four companies, two, Pfizer and Commercial Solvents, were
not originally pharmaceutical companies at all.

The true situation was well summed up by Dr. Norman
Heatley:

> Florey has often been criticised for "giving away to America" a
> project which might have earned this country millions of dollars.
> It is true that huge sums have been made from penicillin, but the
> criticism will not bear examination. In the first place the Oxford
> process for growing the fungus and extracting the penicillin only
> became commercially practicable when the yield had been greatly
> increased by the work at Peoria and elsewhere in America. It is
> doubtful whether useful patents could have been obtained in
> England in 1941 and there was no mechanism by which the Uni-
> versity, for instance, could have assisted. Finally when Florey
> sought high-level advice on the question, he was told authorita-

tively that the patenting of a potentially beneficial medical discovery or invention was against medical ethics and, from that point of view, out of the question.

Fleming obviously leaned strongly toward Florey's traditionalist view on the matter of patents. Speaking at a dinner in his honor in New York in June 1945, he declared: "When the basic information was given free to the world it seems a pity that people here and there should seek to make capital out of what is, after all, a matter of detail."

There were many lessons to be learned from the story of penicillin. Florey and Chain both drew different conclusions from the failure to make penicillin into a profit-winner as well as a life-saver. In Britain and America there were programs, both official and commercial, to advance further into the realm of chemotherapy which penicillin had opened.

Chapter 14
THE LESSONS
OF PENICILLIN

THE LESSONS OF PENICILLIN IN THE U.S.A.

THE CHIEF LESSON that penicillin taught the world was that chemotherapy was a major weapon in the fight against disease; that drugs could be found which could be safely introduced into the body where they would kill invading micro-organisms without killing the patient. Furthermore, penicillin had been found in nature rather than being created by the chemist. It was reasonable to expect, therefore, that there would be other natural substances which would kill germs, including those that penicillin could not affect. Penicillin caused the antibiotic revolution and founded the antibiotic pharmaceutical industry.

The Americans were the quickest to learn this lesson. Indeed they hardly needed to learn it from penicillin for they had nearly reached this point by a different route. American scientists knew, as well as any in Europe, of the long history of "bacterial antagonism"; they knew that many substances were produced by micro-organisms that would kill or stop the growth of bacteria and other germs. One man, in particular, was interested enough in bacterial antagonism to do further work on it. This was Professor Selman A. Waksman of Rutgers University (New Brunswick, N.J.). He had been working as consultant to the Merck Company, which was commercially involved, as Pfizer was, in the production of chemical raw materials by fermentation processes: feeding micro-organisms which produced the desired chemicals as a by-product of their life-cycles. Waksman was basically a soil-microbiologist and particularly interested in the creation of humus by natural methods. One of the organisms most responsible for humus production is the family of molds called streptomycetes, and Waksman duly built up in his Rutgers laboratory one of the world's largest scientific collections of streptomycetes.

This particular family of micro-organisms had figured largely in the world's scientific literature on bacterial antagonism. Waksman became interested in seeing what antibacterial substances he could obtain from his collection of specimens at almost exactly the same time as Florey and Chain decided to look at bacterial antagonism. His program was begun in 1939 in the Department of Microbiology of the New Jersey Agricultural Experimental Station which was part of Rutgers University. Within the next two years he isolated a number of antibacterial substances from his streptomycetes, but all of them were rather toxic to human cells and animals. This emphasizes the importance of the "luck" that penicillin was essentially non-toxic to human cells; it was its non-toxicity that made penicillin the first.

By 1941 Waksman was aware of penicillin in some detail and likewise aware that it would go into production, if possible. Because penicillin seemed active only against Gram-positive organisms, Waksman searched for something that would be active against Gram-negative bacteria.

By 1942 Waksman had isolated an antibiotic substance

(streptothricin) from the organism *Streptomyces lavendulae.* It was fairly stable chemically, easily manageable and it was active against Gram-negative as well as against some Gram-positive organisms. But after this promising start there were disappointments, for streptothricin turned out to be toxic when tested on animals, not frightfully toxic like some of Waksman's earlier discoveries, but too dangerous to be used on humans.

Persistently he went on and by September 1943 he had isolated yet another antibiotic, this time from *Streptomyces griseus.* By January 1944 he was able to announce the discovery of streptomycin, the first broad-spectrum antibiotic, active against a wide variety of organisms both Gram-positive and Gram-negative. Furthermore, clinical trials soon showed that streptomycin was active against the germ causing tuberculosis, *Mycobacterium tuberculosis,* and this, the second useful antibiotic, is still used in treatment of TB.

Virtually every American pharmaceutical company had by now launched massive screening programs in which soil, dust and molds from every part of the world were examined for antibacterial activity. From a sample of soil from a field in Venezuela came an organism which was appropriately christened *Streptomyces venezuelae.* It provided chloramphenicol in 1947, and, when its structure was established in 1949 by the chemists of the Parke Davis and Company, it was found possible to synthesize it. Chloramphenicol thus became the first synthetic antibiotic to be put on the market. Another streptomycete gave the Lederle Laboratories the antibiotic Aureomycin in 1948. Pfizer came up with Terramycin in 1950, again the source being a streptomycete.

There have been many other antibiotics since then, and several have been developed outside the U.S.A. Broadly speaking, the modern antibiotics industry was established by these American companies in the first five years after the end of the war by vigorous searching in the places to which penicillin had pointed the way: the dusty, earthy, moldy corners of the world. Each one of these early antibiotics has also led to the discovery of close relatives or slightly modified descendants. They survive in the marketplace only if they survive in the medical armory because they are more active against some particular germ or group of germs than any of their rivals.

The other chief line of antibiotic research in America was the drive to find a way to synthesize penicillin, a project which was also pursued, though less actively, in Britain. Professor Chain, speaking at the Penicillin "Thirtieth Anniversary Meeting" remembered: "As the structural features of the penicillin molecule slowly came to light, the opinion held by the overwhelming majority of the organic chemists working on this problem was that it would only be a matter of months before the penicillin molecule would be synthesized. I personally never shared this optimistic view and we had some heated arguments in various committees." The problem was, in essence, the closing of the rings of the penicillin molecule's nucleus, those rings that are so easily opened by acid or heat to render penicillin valueless. The job was not done till 1957 when John C. Sheehan at last succeeded after nearly ten years of work in Boston. His eventual success depended upon the discovery of an entirely new family of ring-closing chemicals, a discovery made by chemists working in other fields. Furthermore, Sheehan's work has never led to practical results because the yield of penicillin from his process is so small that no one has seen any way of making it economic in industrial terms.

THE LESSONS OF PENICILLIN IN BRITAIN

In Britain in 1945 the lessons of penicillin seemed at first to be quite different. The affair of the patents was still rankling and the first license fees were being paid to America, despite the dollar shortage, for the recently imported deep-fermentation secrets. Those pharmaceutical companies not involved in deep fermentation were giving up the manufacture of antibiotics completely and hoping to face the economic consequences of the war with different types of products. Very little screening for fresh antibiotics was carried on, though there was still quite an enthusiastic search for methods of synthesizing penicillin.

In Britain it seemed that the administrative structure was at fault. What the country needed was some mechanism by which the products of our university scientists could be brought out of the laboratory and got to the stage of industrial development. The British had seen the research grants from the Office of Scientific Research and Development and the War Production Board in America helping American applied scientists and pharmaceutical companies through those stages of prototype and pilot-plant development. They had seen American chemical-engineering expertise really applied to the production of penicillin, whereas Britain had simply been forced to an ultimately unsatisfactory scaling-up of the laboratory process.

The other wartime British inventions of radar and the jet engine had been developed to the stage of industrial production with complete success. But radar and the jet engine were direct weapons of war; their development from the laboratory into production had been directly financed by the armed services through the various ministries.

And so the post-war Labour government invented an entirely new type of government agency. This was the National Research Development Corporation (notice it is not Research *and* Development). This body, hereinafter called N.R.D.C., was independent of government but financed by the treasury department. Its objective was to take up worthwhile inventions by scientists in the government research establishments (such as the Radar Research Establishment at Malvern), the universities or individual inventors. N.R.D.C. would help with patenting problems and would provide finances for the development of prototypes or for industrial study of the invention right up to the stage where industry was prepared to support the project completely in the usual commercial way.

The legislation setting up the N.R.D.C. was brought before Parliament by the up-and-coming young Labour minister at the Board of Trade, Mr. Harold Wilson. And the N.R.D.C. is still in existence, having been a favored instrument of succeeding Labour governments and having had spells when its role has been reduced when the Conservative party has been in power in Britain. It has found other methods of working as well as those originally laid down for it and is probably best known for its sponsorship of Sir Christopher Cockerell's "Hovercraft" principle. It has developed the basic ideas of air-cushion vehicles into seagoing Hovercraft and the land-borne Hovertrain as well as various methods of industrial load movement.

But the most profitable of all the investments made by the N.R.D.C. in its twenty-five years of history has been its support of a new antibiotic. And in following the development of this new antibiotic in a little detail one can see how the British applied what they considered the further lessons of the penicillin story and how the regrets over what had happened to penicillin drove men to persistence beyond the bounds of commercial wisdom. Yet this un-commercial persistence resulted in vast commercial profits in the end.

This is the story of the antibiotic cephalosporin which is marketed as Ceporin. It begins in the sewers of Sardinia. The man who started it was Professor Giuseppe Brotzu, a biochemist in the Public Health Service at Cagliari. His approach to the problem of finding a new antibiotic seems considerably more elegant, not to say more intelligent, than the vast screening processes favored by U.S. scientists. He wanted particularly to find an antibiotic which would be effective against typhoid; he argued that it was likely to be produced by some organism which either fed on typhoid bacilli or which co-existed with them. The obvious place to find typhoid germs was in the sewers, so he betook himself to the outfall of Cagliari's sewage system at a place called Su Siccu, and started to take samples. In 1945 he found an organism *Cephalosporium acremonium,* a mold which produced in culture a substance that was biologically active against the salmonella organisms which cause typhoid, and was active against other germs as well.

His results were published in the *Journal of the Institute of*

Health of Cagliari, but he knew quite well that there was little chance of his work being noted from such a source. He therefore contacted Dr. H. Blythe Brook, who had been working in Sardinia for the Allied Military Government before the end of the war, when Italy was reduced to the peculiar role of co-belligerent. The two men had met when both were concerned with the public health problems of Sardinia under this rather strange regime. Dr. Blythe Brook was by this time medical officer of health for one of the London boroughs and not in a position to do any research. Instead he brought Professor Brotzu's discovery to the notice of Florey, still at Oxford, and arranged for samples of Brotzu's mold to be sent to Oxford.

Chain had by this time left Oxford (for reasons and with results that will appear in the next chapter). Dr. E.P. Abraham had succeeded to the leadership of the chemists in Florey's department, with the official title of reader in chemical pathology (incidentally, he is still at the Sir William Dunn School of Pathology with the rank, now, of professor). His assistant in the work that was about to start on the cephalosporia was Dr. G.G.F. Newton. Florey had already been made Sir Howard Florey, and was eventually to become Lord Florey.

The very first experiments carried out on Brotzu's mold at Oxford confirmed his findings. There was indeed an antibacterial substance produced by the organism, but detailed examination showed that this antibacterial consisted of three different substances. They were called cephalosporins on the analogy of the production of the word penicillin. There was cephalosporin P and cephalosporin N and a third (minor and for the moment unidentified) component.

Cephalosporin P was soon shown to be active against only a fairly small range of micro-organisms. Yet it was of considerable interest to the chemists, at least academically, because it was, although an antibiotic, a steroid which had never been seen before. Cephalosporin N was much more interesting from the point of view of a possible commercial antibiotic. It was fairly powerful, active against many of the Gram-negative bacteria which were untouched by penicillin, and at this stage of the story the great range of American-produced antibiotics which were also active against Gram-negative organisms had not yet flooded the market.

At this point the Medical Research Council's Antibiotic Research Station at Clevedon was called in to help. Clevedon, which had been the Royal Navy's penicillin production establishment during the war, was itself part of the British reaction to the penicillin story. It had been equipped with a fermentation plant on a semi-industrial scale precisely to carry out research into fermentation processes and their effects on antibiotic production because it was clearly in this field that the Americans had had such advantage when it came to producing penicillin. Clevedon was set to work to produce considerable quantities of cephalosporin N and P so that the Oxford chemists would have a reasonable amount of material to work on, and would not have to suffer the delays caused by lack of material which had so affected the penicillin work seven years earlier.

Backed by a fairly large production of the mold and its products at Clevedon, the Oxford chemists settled down to a broad attack on the cephalosporins as an academic program primarily, but also with the added interest of finding that cephalosporin N was rather effective against typhoid germs and accounted for Brotzu's original findings. As academics they were interested rather than disappointed when it turned out that cephalosporin N was in fact a penicillin. It had the 6APA nucleus of the penicillin molecules, and it only differed from the substances produced by the penicillium molds in the structure of its side-chain. Furthermore, it turned out that cephalosporin N was identical with another new antibiotic, Synnematin B, which had been discovered by a Federal Research Laboratory and developed by the Abbott Company (Laboratories) in the U.S.A. Abbott had also found that its Synnematin was active against typhoid germs and had actually manufactured 1000 grams of and sent it to South America where it was tested on, and used to control, an epidemic of typhoid. This penicillin-Synnematin-cephalosporin N was overtaken by the more powerful antibiotics produced by other U.S. companies and disappears from the story. The Oxford chemists proceeded quietly with their academic program of research into the interesting products of the cephalosporia molds.

At this stage the third, and minor, component of Brotzu's original antibacterial substance began to attract notice. It was present as a very small proportion of impurity in the partially purified cephalosporin N. Clevedon was sending cephalosporin N in reasonable quantities to Oxford during the studies that showed cephalosporin N was a penicillin. It was almost certainly present in larger quantities in the Clevedon fermentation of cephalosporium and some of it was removed during the partial purification of cephalosporin N.

Abraham and Newton eventually isolated this minor component and called it cephalosporin C. Chemical studies showed that it was not a penicillin and it eventually turned out to be a true cephalosporin, something new to science. Even more interesting, the first studies of its biological activity showed that although it was much less active against germs than the normal penicillins then widely available, it was not destroyed by the strains of germs that were resistant to penicillin. Indeed, it could kill the penicillin-resistant bacteria.

The importance of this discovery requires a short digression. From the earliest days of this research it had been known that some strains of bacteria were not killed by the drug even though they were of types that normally fell easy victims to penicillin. This was essentially different from the phenomenon of the types of germs which had never been affected by penicillin, such as the Gram-negative bacteria. In these penicillin-resistant strains there was a mutation, a variation from their family norm, which enabled them to resist and destroy penicillin. In the types of germ which were never affected by penicillin we have seen that this invulnerability to the antibiotic is primarily because they have a different cell-wall structure from the Gram-positive bacteria. In the penicillin-resistant strains, the cell wall was just the same as in their vulnerable brothers, but the resistant strains had the ability to produce a chemical, an enzyme, called penicillinase which could destroy the activity of the penicillin molecule by breaking open one of its ring structures. (For the record: it is known now that certain types of bacteria which are not affected by penicillin also produce penicillinase naturally.)

As the wide, often indiscriminate, use of penicillin spread around the post-war world those strains of germs vulnerable to penicillin were very nearly wiped out. This gave the resistant strains of the same germs a chance to spread and increase their area of existence, in exactly the same way we believe evolution and "survival of the fittest" normally works. At the worst times and places penicillin-resistant germs caused as many as eighty percent of infections by staphylococci and streptococci in some British and U.S. hospitals. It seemed at one time that penicillin would simply fall into disuse, especially when it was discovered that bacteria do have a process, similar to the sexual process, by which a penicillin-resistant bacterium can transfer the genetic material which gives it the power to manufacture penicillinase to another bacterium which did not originally have this power.

(It should be mentioned that Fleming went back to research work on penicillin after his first experience of its curative powers in 1942 and, among his many claims to a place in the penicillin story, not the least is his firm establishment of the existence of naturally occurring resistant strains of germs.)

The extremely serious full development of penicillin-resistant strains of bacteria had not been reached by the time of the discovery of the power of cephalosporin C to kill penicillin-resistant cocci. But it was already looming as a problem serious enough to make this discovery of great interest and to raise the possibility that cephalosporin C might become an antibiotic of great value. Interest in it increased as Abraham and Newton showed that it was even less toxic to animals than penicillin; that it was soluble in water and not easily destroyed by acid, so that it could, as a drug, be administered by mouth and be able to cross the wall of the human gut into the bloodstream.

There were two problems facing cephalosporin C at this time in its progress toward becoming a commercial drug. First, despite its admirable properties it was nothing like as active as the penicillins and other antibiotics and would have to be used in huge doses. Second, it could only be produced in extremely small quantities; it was still a minor component in the brew at Clevedon. The time scale was also becoming very long: Brotzu had made his original discovery in 1945; work at Oxford had started on a fair level in 1947; it was now 1954 and no extra money had yet been put into the project, it had all been borne on the normal academic budgets of Oxford and Clevedon.

However the N.R.D.C., in accordance with its terms of reference, had been steadily patenting Abraham's results ever since he had started working on cephalosporin C in 1951. By 1955 when Abraham had definitely established the chemical structure of the molecule as a two-ring structure, similar to but definitely different from penicillin and with two side-chains instead of one, the N.R.D.C. decided it was time to call in the help of industry.

The proposal that N.R.D.C. took to the pharmaceutical companies was that they should join in the development of this possibly interesting antibiotic, and that they should bring their expertise in chemical engineering and fermentation to bear on the production problem. In exchange, of course, for eventual rights in the developed product. A target figure of the production of 100 grams of cephalosporin C was set up and several British pharmaceutical companies agreed to look at the problem.

But progress was slow. The usual industrial "wisdom" failed to produce greater amounts of cephalosporin C and the yield remained desperately low. Some companies soon lost interest; one in particular decided to concentrate all its efforts in the field of developing the first oral contraceptives. And it was in fact the M.R.C. scientists at Clevedon who achieved the big step forward when they found that a mutant of Brotzu's original *Cephalosporium acremonium* seemed to prefer to make cephalosporin C rather than the other constituents. Suddenly

252 IN SEARCH OF PENICILLIN

yields changed from "trace quantities" to "significant." These
yields were still not of a size that could possibly be commercially viable, but they did enable the target figure of 100 grams
to be produced, and that in turn enabled a major scientific
program to be launched at Oxford.

The immediate results of this program brought another
time of near despair in the development of the new antibiotic.
Although the increased quantity of cephalosporin now available made it possible to confirm all the previous claims for its
desirability (its action against penicillin-resistant germs, its
non-toxicity, its solubility and its acid-resistance), it exhibited
something known only too well in the pharmaceutical industry. While it would work well against germs in laboratory glassware, its activity in the living body was very much reduced,
indeed it would barely work at all.

It was now 1958, and already it was known that the research
team at Beecham's had opened the way, in theory at least, to
the creation of large numbers of semi-synthetic penicillins
which could presumably be "tailored" to do any particular job
of attacking disease organisms (this development is the subject
of the next chapter). On the other hand, they had not yet put
on the market any semi-synthetic penicillin which was either
active against Gram-negative organisms or against penicillin-
resistant organisms. It was also becoming plain that bacteria
resistant to the post-penicillin antibiotics developed in America—resistant to Aureomycin, streptomycin, the tetracyclines
and so on—were gradually becoming more and more of a
medical problem. There could still be a place for cephalosporin C, but it is most unlikely that its development would have
been pursued any further at this time if purely commercial
motives had been the only ones.

It is at this point that the reason for describing the development of something that is not penicillin becomes most relevant. It was just here that the British desire to "atone" for their
failure to develop penicillin to commercial success played its
most vital part.

"At this stage the whole development of cephalosporin C

was poised vitally between failure and success," according to Dr. Basil A.J. Bard, of N.R.D.C., who was involved in the cephalosporin story throughout much of this crucial time. Senior executives of the Glaxo Company (which eventually brought the antibiotic to the market) have told me that, though their company's motives were purely commercial, they were aware of what they named "the American penicillin syndrome" time and again in their dealings with scientists and the officials of N.R.D.C. and even of the central government. And everybody I have questioned who was involved in the development of cephalosporin C, when asked if any one man was responsible for keeping the project going, replied: "Florey."

From the scientific point of view the next move was fairly obvious. They would remove cephalosporin's natural side-chain, or at least one of them, and replace it with the side-chain that made ordinary penicillin G so effective. In the laboratory this worked, though it was quite plain that the laboratory methods of doing it could not be applied industrially. It was not as simple as dealing with penicillin because cephalosporin had two side-chains, and one tended to mask the effect of the other. Furthermore, the interaction between different side-chains seemed to be illogical. It proved impossible to predict in the usual way what any one side-chain would do in the presence of any other. In addition to this it was found that animal livers would neatly and rapidly split off some of the side-chains that the chemists had so laboriously stuck on. This accounted for some of the early variations of cephalosporin C being found effective against germs in the test-tube but not working satisfactorily in living bodies.

Nevertheless, sufficient progress was made for a number of further pharmaceutical companies to become interested in cephalosporin, including some U.S. companies. And here the N.R.D.C. policy of patenting Abraham's early discoveries paid off. They were able to make license agreements that contained clauses demanding that techniques and knowledge acquired by these companies in any joint research projects on cephalosporin would have to be fed back to the patent-holder,

N.R.D.C. The patent position had one weakness, it was now ten years since Abraham's earliest work on cephalosporin C, and the patents, in the usual way, only provided fifteen years' protection.

The testing of large numbers of variations of side-chains on the basic nucleus of the cephalosporin molecule was work for the research departments of pharmaceutical firms, rather than for a comparatively small university laboratory. The story now passes to the Glaxo Company, for it was in its laboratories that the compound code-numbered 87/4 emerged. This substance is 7-[(2-thienyl)acetamido]-3-(1-pyridylmethyl)-3-cephem-4-carboxylic acid betaine.

First tests showed that, in the laboratory, it was active against a wide spectrum of infective organisms. The story can be followed from the official record of the Glaxo Company, Glaxo Volume 28:

> Now arose the question, is it active in vivo? Mice experimentally infected with a wide range of test organisms showed it was, with curative doses down to practicable low levels. Was it active in other animal species? Rats and rabbits were also protected. Rabbits, infected with virulent strains of staphylococci, and allowed to deteriorate without treatment until they were acutely ill and within a few hours of death, were snatched back to health with small doses. What about resistance to penicillinase? Cephaloridine [the name finally given to 87/4] was found to be over four thousand times as resistant as benzylpenicillin to penicillinase, and it was fully active both in vitro and in vivo against penicillin-resistant strains of *Staphylococcus aureus*.

So cephaloridine had all the desirable qualities shown by its ancestor, cephalosporin C. But might it do more harm than good? The Glaxo Volume again:

> Toxicologists are dedicated men with sad eyes and a sense of foreboding. To them all new drugs are nowadays suspected as potential killers, or derangers of the mind, or distorters of the fetus. Pregnancy is merely an enforced period of drug denial. Into this atmosphere the new cephalosporin had to go—to be sub-

jected to an exhaustive series of acute and subacute and chronic toxicity testing; to test for any effects on respiration or circulation or excretory, central nervous and reproductive functions; and all these in several animal species. Cephaloridine has emerged with a clean bill of health; it is apparently a very safe drug, at any rate at dose levels likely to be used therapeutically.

And as a final bonus it turned out that cephaloridine inflicted remarkably little local pain when injected intramuscularly. This is even more extraordinary since cephalosporin C, and several other cephalosporins which had been tested, caused considerable pain when injected.

After that it was a straight problem of getting cephaloridine into production and onto the market. This is a rather brutal summation of three years' work by biologists, bacteriologists, chemical engineers and marketing men. But it must suffice here. There is only one point in these three years that is relevant to our story. It concerns the method of stripping off the natural side-chains of cephalosporin C in order that the more effective side-chains of cephaloridine could be attached to the nucleus. The best method of doing this on an industrial scale was discovered in the research laboratories of Eli Lilly and Co. in the U.S.A. But under the N.R.D.C. license agreements this know-how had to be fed back to Britain and could be made available to Glaxo when they came to the manufacturing process.

Cephaloridine was marketed (as Ceporin) in 1964. Glaxo had spent £2 million in their ten years of work on the drug, and they recouped their investment by 1970. Other antibiotics of the same family are expected to be produced, so that will provide a further payoff. N.R.D.C. invested £60,000 in the development and patenting of cephaloridine over the nineteen years between its discovery and its marketing. But license fees under the many patents now form the biggest single source of income for this semi-official corporation, and these incomes, much of it in dollars, can be re-invested in new inventions. Glaxo also earns a very large amount of dollar and foreign currency from direct sales of the drug.

It is, of course, a matter of personal political view whether one regards N.R.D.C. as being a viable and worthwhile agency, whether it is a desirable political invention. In describing its role in the development of Ceporin it has undoubtedly appeared in the best possible light, for this particular development is its greatest commercial triumph. There are many who feel that the development of inventions should be left strictly to private industry, and that an invention which cannot obtain support in the marketplace cannot really be worthwhile. On the other hand, a number of countries have followed the British example and set up agencies or corporations similar to N.R.D.C.

But these arguments are not strictly relevant to the story of penicillin. The point is simply that both N.R.D.C. and the new antibiotic it helped to bring to the continuing battle against disease and sickness are the direct consequences of what happened in the development of penicillin and the commercial and psychological scars that penicillin left in Britain in 1945.

Chapter 15
PENICILLIN
AS YOU LIKE IT

THE GREATEST PLEASURE in writing the story of penicillin lies in the fact that history presents such magnificent examples of the classical principles of dramatic unity. The same characters keep cropping up in the story, in a way which no modern writer of fiction would dare to impose upon his public.

Two more chapters of the story of penicillin revolve around a character who entered the picture at a very early stage, Sir Ernst Boris Chain. He drew entirely different lessons from the early history of penicillin than those drawn by other people.

In 1944 and 1945 as the structure of penicillin became clear he did not believe that penicillin would soon be synthesized. But he admits to being almost alone in this belief. In 1963 he said:

> On the other hand many scientists in both industrial and academic laboratories took the view that a synthesis of penicillin

could be achieved which would solve all production troubles, and a very large effort was expended in this direction. A few hundred chemists were engaged in this effort for a period of more than five years. Estimating the annual cost of each chemist, plus research expenses, modestly at £5000, this effort to synthesise the penicillin molecule, which proved a failure, has cost a total of several million pounds—yet another good example . . . of the professional hazards encountered by the pharmaceutical industry.

Nor did Chain think highly of the vast screening programs for the new antibiotics launched by the American pharmaceutical industry in those same years: "If one considers the immense effort which was expended in the search for new antibiotics of clinical usefulness, the result must be considered as meagre. Many hundreds of people participated in the effort, and hundreds of millions of dollars were spent for screening micro-organisms from the air, the earth and water, with the result of a dozen or so of antibiotics of clinical importance."

Chain's reaction to the penicillin story was different. He believed that the Oxford work had been unnecessarily held up because of the lack of large-scale fermentation equipment which would have provided the scientists with sufficient material for experiments. He demanded pilot plant fermentation tanks on a semi-industrial scale. He did not get it at Oxford or at any other British university.

So Chain parted from Florey and Oxford and went off to Rome, where the Institute of Health invited him to set up a biochemical department equipped on the scale he wanted. In biochemical terms what Chain wanted to do was to experiment further with the development of new forms of penicillin. He believed that adding new nutrients, or precursors, to the medium in which the molds grew would enable the molds to produce new penicillins with new forms of side-chain. Even if the new penicillins produced by biosynthesis (manufacture by living bodies) were not entirely satisfactory in themselves, perhaps they could be modified by further chemical reactions outside the fermenters into useful new drugs. He was not the only person to adopt this approach, but by the time his plant at the Institute of Health in Rome was fully active he was thinking that on these lines there was an approach to the now threatening penicillin-resistant strains of bacteria. In particular he thought, on the basis of general biochemical principles, that a variation of penicillin G—an aminobenzylpenicillin—could be provided by fermentation and would have a side-chain that could be manipulated in such a way as to provide protection against penicillinase, produced by penicillin-resistant strains of germs.

Whether or not it was frustration that drove Chain to leave Oxford, it was certainly frustration that eventually brought the Beecham Group into contact with him. Beecham was a group founded on the success of the Pills and Powders produced in the nineteenth century by Doctor Beecham. The company developed into the twentieth century primarily as a manufacturer of proprietary medicines (medicines in Britain that can be advertised publicly and sold over the chemists' shop counters without a doctor's prescription, for what is now called self-medication). In the 1920s and 1930s the company's management was highly competent, in commercial terms, and they expanded into the fields of toiletries, cosmetics and food. Toothpaste and haircream were among the best-known products to come into the company's product lines. A small "ethical" chemical company was also acquired (ethical chemicals or drugs being those that are not advertised publicly and which require a doctor's prescription before they can be purchased).

In the later years of the war Beecham became very anxious to enter the antibiotics field as it saw how important penicillin was becoming. But it was rebuffed by the Ministry of Supply when it sought a license to start manufacturing penicillin in 1945. Despite a number of efforts to get into penicillin in other ways, the only success the group could obtain was a contract to develop penicillin-containing pastilles for the treatment of infections of the mouth. The contract came from the Royal Air Force, the penicillin was manufactured by other firms and Beecham's part was simply the incorporation of the drug into satisfactory gelatin-based capsules.

Meanwhile, the production of penicillin increased apace.

Peace brought with it the prospect of widespread civilian use of penicillin and there were rumors of penicillin-containing toothpastes, lipsticks and haircreams, so that Beecham's traditional markets were threatened. Company executives were soon in the U.S.A. to try to obtain licenses on penicillin-manufacturing processes, particularly from Pfizer. The group's (unpublished) account records: "A discussion with the Chairman of that company revealed that there was no intention of parting with any information on the processes to any other company."

In Britain the Therapeutic Substances Act was in the offing (it became law in 1947) restricting the sale of penicillin to registered pharmacists' shops and on doctor's prescription only, so that penicillin-containing toiletries never came on the market. But Beecham Research Laboratories Limited had come into existence and opened a new research establishment at Brockham Park, a country house near Dorking to the south of London. The official opening was performed by Sir Alexander Fleming, but for the first years of its existence the new laboratory was mostly concerned with revivifying the group's more traditional products.

By 1952, however, the group was looking at penicillin again. The idea was to do some research on ways in which penicillin G could be treated so that higher concentrations of the drug could be got into the bloodstream and system when it was taken by mouth. Talks took place with the U.S. pharmaceutical company, Bristol-Myers. It advised Beecham against going into penicillin production because, although world production of penicillin G was still increasing, this was largely accounted for by the start of manufacture in so many countries outside the U.S.A. and Britain. There was, in fact, overproduction in America and the price of penicillin G had fallen so much that a dose of the drug was worth very little more than the ampule used to contain it, in money terms at least.

But in 1953, penicillin V came into the picture, originally discovered by the Eli Lilly Co. in the U.S. in 1945 and rediscovered in Austria five years later. The important thing about penicillin V was that, though not so active against some germs as penicillin G in the absolute sense, it could be taken by mouth and pass into the bloodstream in quite high concentrations. From 1954 it became the penicillin of choice when oral administration was required. And so another effort by Beecham to enter the penicillin business came to nothing.

It was in 1955 that the group sought the advice of Professor Chain, for reasons that had nothing to do with penicillin but were relevant to aspects of the history of penicillin in a most curious coincidence. Beecham had been expanding very happily in all its other fields of activity despite its lack of progress in the penicillin field. It had become probably the world's largest user of tartaric acid at the same time as, by development of its pre-war fermentation method, Pfizer had become the only large-scale supplier in the world. Potentially this put Beecham in a vulnerable position. Beecham wondered whether it should try to find other industrial processes for synthesizing tartaric acid, which laboratory chemistry had shown to be possible. The group's scientific consultant, Sir Charles Dodds, advised them to get in touch with Chain who was doing studies in his Rome fermentation plants on the production of citric acid by fermentation.

A meeting with Chain was arranged for a day in May 1955, when he was to be in London to give a lecture at the Royal Society. At this meeting it was suggested that some of the Beecham research men should come out to Rome to learn about Chain's fermentation techniques with a view to starting some of their own research into the tartaric-acid problem. It was also mentioned that the group was still interested in finding a way into the antibiotics field.

In a series of further meetings through the summer of 1955 a more exciting plan was worked out: Chain became officially consultant to the group; a large microbiological research project was to be added at the Brockham Park laboratories with pilot-plant-size fermentation equipment; a small group was to go out from Brockham Park to work with Chain in

Rome; the chief drive would be toward producing new types of penicillin on the lines Chain proposed; and there would be longer term work on the problems of tartaric acid.

In the first half of 1956 Beecham sent Dr. George N. Rolinson (a microbiologist), Mr. Ralph Batchelor (a biochemist) and Dr. Merfyn Richards (a mycologist) to work with Chain. The building of the microbiological laboratories and pilot plant facilities was put in hand at Brockham Park, with the director, Dr. John Farquharson, in charge. Of the staff already at Brockham Park the two chemists, Dr. F. Peter Doyle and Dr. John H.C. Nayler, were also to play large parts in the coming events.

The essential feature of that year's work in Rome was that two of the men—with Chain directing, and working with the Italian scientists of the Institute of Health—managed to find a fermentation process which produced the p-aminobenzyl-penicillin. Chain thought this would be a good starting material for further work, and they produced it with fairly satisfactory yields. Some was sent back to England and Beecham made thirty new varieties of penicillin, though none of these were of commercial value.

By the following year, in May 1957, the scientists were back in England and started the same process in the pilot-plant fermenters at Brockham Park. In the course of getting the production going, naturally there was a lot of measurement of what was being produced. The production of penicillin can be measured in various ways. There is the biological assay method: essentially the one Heatley devised (Oxford, 1940) in which the area of germs destroyed by the penicillin in a culture plate is the vital measurement. Also by this time there were chemical measurements available; notably, one in which penicillin was reacted with a substance called hydroxylamine and the amount of penicillin from the reaction measured. Also available: a method of assaying the amount of penicillin present in a mixture by using penicillinase to destroy it, and measuring the amount of acid liberated by the destruction.

But in May 1957, the workers at Brockham Park noticed that they were getting different results from their chemical and biological tests, just as they had earlier in Rome. The chemical measurements showed that a certain amount of penicillin was present in one of their brews, but the biological tests showed that the same brew had distinctly less penicillin as judged by its activity against germs. In principle this sort of difference had long been known among research laboratories engaged in antibiotic research. But here the difference seemed very marked and it seemed to become more obvious in brews to which no side-chain precursor material had been added.

The two men who had been in Rome had noticed something of the same sort when they had been working there, but the discrepancies had been small and they had been too busy working with p-aminobenzylpenicillin to pursue it. Now they discussed it again, and this time with the chemists. It was suggested there might be some material in the brew which was chemically a penicillin (because it was destroyed by penicillinase) but which did not work as an antibiotic against germs. Why should there be more of this material, though, when no extra side-chain precursor material had been added to the brew? Rolinson and Batchelor came up with the exciting suggestion that the unknown material might be the nucleus of penicillin without any side-chain attached to it: pure 6-APA. No one can now remember at just which of the innumerable discussions this possibility was first mentioned.

It was the chemists at Brockham Park who suggested an experiment to prove that there was pure 6-APA in the brews. They proposed to add to the brew the ordinary chemical that made the side-chain of one of the usual penicillins (G or V) in such a way that it would join on to the 6-APA, if that were indeed present, and produce a normal antibiotic penicillin. They did this and, sure enough, the chemical and biological assays came into agreement. This did not prove the case, but it made it seem very likely that pure 6-APA was present.

When this result was reported to Dr. Farquharson he immediately ordered that all other work should be stopped to follow up this lead. The first thing must be to find out if 6-APA was really present and to prove it beyond doubt. Because, if it was indeed so, they had an amazing situation on their hands. If they could produce 6-APA and extract it from the brew they could add any side-chains they wished. They would no longer be tied to using only the substances the mold would accept and use. Thousands of new pencillins could be made at will. New molecules could be produced that would meet specific medical needs: antibiotics could be made to meet even resistant germs, Gram-negative or Gram-positive; virtually anything could be done. The horizon seemed limitless.

The way in which the Beecham men proved their case was extremely neat. It depended on paper chromatography, a development of the technique used by Chain and Abraham in purifying the first penicillin in Oxford, in which a spot of a mixture of substances is placed at one end of a strip of absorbent paper (rather like blotting paper) and then a solvent is allowed to diffuse through the paper from that same end of the strip. When everything is chosen correctly all the different substances in the original mixture will travel different distances along the strip of paper and become separated from each other so that each one can later be identified. If the research involves an antibiotic the strips of paper can afterward be laid on the agar in a Petri dish and germs will be prevented from growing around the place on the paper containing the antibiotic. This is a variation of Fleming's ditch test.

The Beecham team prepared six strips of chromatography paper and a large dish of agar seeded with germ organisms. On the first strip they put their brew, suspected of containing both penicillins and 6-APA, and ran the solvent through it. On the plate it produced inhibition of germs in a big patch right near the middle, showing that penicillins were indeed present. On the second strip they put their brew after it had been treated with butyl acetate, which would extract the penicillins as amyl acetate had done in the earliest work but would not extract the 6-APA because of its chemical structure. This strip showed no zones of inhibition of germs, which implied that the mystery structure might be there; but if so it was not antibiotic.

The third strip was treated in the same way as the second, removing the antibiotics, but before placing it on the agar they performed the same trick as in their earlier suggestive but not final experiment: they added the side-chain of penicillin G in reactive form which would join with 6-APA, if it was present, to give penicillin G which they could identify. And, sure enough, a zone of inhibition appeared on the agar plate, not near the middle of the strip but near the start. This proved that the original brew contained a substance that had not got the same structure as a full penicillin because it did not run so far down the strip as a penicillin, but which could form an antibiotic when a side-chain was added to it.

Strip number four received a similar application but the brew had been treated with penicillinase before being applied. There were no zones of inhibition under this strip when it was put on the germ-coated agar plate, therefore all the antibiotics produced on the previous strips must have had the structures of penicillins. Therefore the mystery substance must have a structure of the penicillin-nucleus type. Strip five had the brew put on it after the acetate treatment had removed all the full penicillins, but the side-chain material had been added before the chromatography had been started. This showed an inhibition area at exactly the same level as the inhibition produced by the natural penicillins on strip one; therefore the new antibiotic made with the mystery substance was a true penicillin. Therefore the mystery substance must be the nucleus of the penicillin molecule, which could be turned into an antibiotic penicillin by having a side-chain added. This meant there was pure 6-APA in the original brew.

The sixth strip simply had ordinary penicillin G put on it before chromatography and this produced inhibition at the same level as strips one and five. This was a control for the rest of the experiment and checked that all the inhibitions at this level were indeed being produced by penicillin types of substances.

It did not prove easy to separate the 6-APA from the brew, but the problem was eventually solved. In the long run two different industrial-scale processes were developed to produce 6-APA. Enough material was available for the chemists to test a wide variety of side-chains in order to find which would give useful new variants of the original antibiotic. These would be the new semi-synthetic penicillins.

For the Beecham Group as a commercial unit the problems and prospects seemed enormous. Beecham had this to itself, it seemed, but the amount of work involved seemed colossal: adding new side-chains to the penicillin nucleus, finding which ones produced drugs of more value than those already on the market, testing out the hopefuls and producing the winners for a world market. Beecham also had to invest in the building of the equipment to produce 6-APA in bulk. It decided to go into partnership in both research and production with their old American friends, the Bristol-Myers Company.

The approach to Bristol was made in a confidential letter to a top executive giving rough details of Beecham's discovery and the immediate follow-up work, which assured Bristol that the job really could be done. This gentleman replied in a rather guarded and noncommittal letter that arrived in England on January 6, 1959. A few hours later highly enthusiastic cablegrams started arriving at Beecham from the same source. The writer of the original letter had not first consulted the scientific staff at Bristol's laboratories at Syracuse. Once the scientists had seen Beecham's evidence they realized what it meant and changed the executive's attitude at speed. Later that month the British scientists announced their major results and their vital discoveries in the scientific journals and then to the mass media. It made a world-wide story, for its implications were obvious: a wide variety of new penicillins could eventually be made.

The British had taken good care of their patent protection this time. They were perhaps slightly lucky here. It turned out that Sheehan (who was, by chance, a consultant to Bristol) had produced a little 6-APA along with many impurities in the course of his route to the complete synthesis of penicillin. There had also been claims by two Japanese groups, Kato in

1953 and Murao in 1955, to have produced 6-APA in fermentation processes. Luckily for Beecham the Japanese work had turned out to be non-reproducible in other laboratories; Chain, for instance, in Rome had failed to get similar results when using their methods. The Beecham men had not, in fact, read of the Japanese work when they performed their crucial experiments. A whole string of patents in Britain and other countries started to be filed (and many to be granted) on 6-APA and the many hundreds of penicillins that could be made by adding side-chains to it. The first application went in as early as August 2, 1957.

The first of the new semi-synthetic penicillins went on the market in America and Britain as early as November 1959. Its official name was phenethecillin. It was a penicillin that could be taken by mouth and gave better levels of antibiotic in the blood (it was more efficiently absorbed into the system) than penicillin V. This was done somewhat at the insistence of Bristol. The company was anxious to market the first semi-synthetic product that showed any reasonable advantage over the existing natural penicillins. There was a good deal of jostling on the starting line even then, with rival companies sending special envoys to Washington in an attempt to see Bristol's official New Drug Application. A paragraph appeared in the *Wall Street Journal* claiming that this particular penicillin was a Pfizer invention. This forced Bristol to make a public scientific announcement about the drug before the company was completely ready to market it. Professor Stewart has this to say: "The therapeutic advantages of these compounds [phenethecillin and its immediate successors] were and are hypothetical, depending entirely upon improved absorption at the expense of intrinsic antibacterial activity. In scientific medical circles, the advent of phenethecillin as the first offspring of the new biosyntheses was something of an anticlimax and the reception was correspondingly lukewarm. With expectation in the air, and in the scientific press, better things had been awaited." Sales, however, were more satisfactory than the scientific reception.

But there was no doubt of the importance, significance and value of the semi-synthetic penicillins that followed. The two major achievements have been penicillins which are not only resistant to penicillinase themselves but also kill the penicillin-resistant germs, and penicillins—at long last—which are effective against Gram-negative organisms, the first wide-spectrum penicillins.

The two main broad-spectrum penicillins are called ampicillin and carbenicillin. There is no doubt of their importance, even if judged only by the way they have swept into the market. They also have considerable theoretical importance by showing that it is indeed possible to find side-chains that can be attached to the 6-APA nucleus to give penicillins having the ability to attack both Gram-positive and Gram-negative organisms.

Perhaps even more valuable was the production of, first, methicillin and then the family of drugs called isoxazolyl-penicillins. These are penicillins that resist the attacks of penicillinase. In principle they do so by having a side-chain which "covers" the weak point in the structure of the nucleus where it is vulnerable to penicillinase. Furthermore, these new man-made drugs can kill the organisms which produced penicillinase. So the problem of the penicillin-resistant germs can at least be met. And there is the promise that if further organisms arise which are resistant even to these new semi-synthetic forms of the drug then even further penicillins can be designed to meet the new threat.

Incidentally, one of the definitions of penicillin in the British Therapeutic Substances Act was that it was "rendered inactive by penicillinase." There had, therefore, to be a legal change to allow the first penicillinase-resistant penicillin, methicillin, to be introduced to the medical armory.

We are living in a new, or second, era of the penicillin revolution. The first revolution wrought by penicillin was to establish the concept of chemotherapy. The second revolution is to open the possibility of chemotherapy being able to adapt itself by producing new products to meet the adaptations nature produces in the micro-organisms.

Professor Stewart has provided the best summing-up of this stage of the development of penicillin: "The story is a minor classic of the circumstances which engender scientific progress; the sound plan for research, the competent all-round team, the probing of a significant anomaly, the good idea, the quick exploitation, and, by no means least, the moral and material support of management and advisers. As with penicillin G, it is a story of purposeful teamwork between industry, hospitals and academic departments, and it is a story worth repeating, for there has been no better road as yet to the cure of disease by medicine."

Chapter 16
PENICILLIN ALLERGY

FROM THE VERY START of the development of semi-synthetic penicillins it had been hoped that it would be possible to produce a family of antibiotics which would not cause the allergic reactions associated with the original natural penicillins. Although the manufacturers of semi-synthetic antibiotics claim that they have made progress toward this end, it is quite clear that no completely non-allergic penicillin has yet appeared on the market. And recent research into the problem of penicillin allergy has shown that the whole situation is much more complicated than had been originally supposed, although the clinical difficulties of dealing with those patients who suffer from penicillin-sensitiveness have been much relieved.

As soon as large-scale clinical tests with penicillin began, back in 1942, it became clear that a number of individuals could not tolerate the new drug. They were either naturally sensitive to it or rapidly became so after the first treatment. Penicillin allergy showed as urticaria (the outbreak of rashes or spots) or as angioedema (tightness of the chest, difficulty in breathing and asthma-like symptoms). In a very few extreme cases individuals who had been sensitized by one treatment with penicillin suffered from anaphylactic shock when they received a further dose of the antibiotic. In some cases they died, especially if immediate up-to-date hospital treatment was not available.

If a drug were to be developed nowadays with these allergic side-effects the U.S. Food and Drug Administration, the Medicines Commission in Britain and comparable bodies in other countries would almost certainly refuse to allow it to be marketed. But penicillin was the first of the antibiotics, and we have seen how astounded were the doctors of the 1940 era with the drug's "miraculous" cures. The problem of reaction seemed slight compared with the usefulness of the treatment.

The first official reports on penicillin allergy were published in America by the National Research Council Division of Medical Sciences Committee on Chemotherapeutic and Other Agents in 1943. The earliest estimates suggested that penicillin allergy was found in approximately one patient in a hundred. Later studies, mostly in America, where penicillin was at first more available, suggested different figures: some were as high as five people in a hundred, others less than one in a hundred.

With thirty years' experience of the use of penicillin behind us, the best estimate is that approximately two people in a hundred will show signs of allergic reaction when treated with penicillin. But this fairly simple statement hides the real problems.

The most urgent of these problems, clinically, is the possibility that any one of the patients sensitive to penicillin may die of anaphylactic shock when given a later dose of the antibiotic. People who have shown themselves sensitive to penicillin are usually given a disk to wear or a card to carry which warns doctors of the possible danger of treating them with the drug.

It is usually sufficient to prescribe some other antibiotic. But there are certain diseases, particularly chest conditions, in which the use of continuous penicillin therapy is desirable, even though the patient has shown sensitivity to the drug. There is no test which will conclusively show what will happen when such an individual is given more penicillin. In extreme cases the doctors simply have to administer the antibiotic in the hospital with a full range of emergency equipment standing ready for use in case the patient goes into shock.

Anaphylactic shock is a medical mystery. It has been known since the very earliest days of immunology, in the time of Pasteur. What happens is that an individual (animal or human) when attacked by, or treated with, a substance which normally causes the standard immune protective reaction, manufactures an unusually large amount of a rather rare antibody called IgE (immunoglobulin E) which is specific to the particular substance which has invaded the body. Any later challenge by the same substance will cause that particular IgE to bind onto the mast-cells and release huge quantities of histamine from these cells. The histamine produces the symptoms of shock and may lower the blood pressure so much as to cause death.

No one has discovered why any particular individual should have such an unusual reaction to one specific challenging substance. The variety of substances which can cause anaphylactic shock or hypersensitivity on the part of the individual is legion. When the hypersensitivity reaction occurs the action of IgE on mast-cells remains shrouded in mystery. Even the role of the mast-cells in the body is not generally agreed upon although it is known that one of their functions is the large-scale manufacture of histamines.

Most doctors, nowadays, would be prepared to accept the statement that penicillin and the other early antibiotics were over-prescribed and used indiscriminately in the treatment of minor ailments where their use was often unnecessary. This has led to the devaluation of many of the early antibiotics through unnecessary exposure of patients to antibiotics in such quantities that allergic sensitivity has been induced. For instance, one of the early studies (which revealed how widespread were the cases of anaphylactic reactions to penicillin) described a fifteen-year-old New York girl in the late 1950s who had been given penicillin injections for "pain in the right knee after a fall" and also for "ear pain."

It is probable that many people who believe that they are allergic or sensitive to penicillin, and who therefore pose an extra problem when they arrive in the doctor's surgery, do not have any real immunological problem. The symptoms known as "ampicillin rash" or "five-day rash" are probably not an allergic reaction at all in many of the people who have suffered from them. A recent report by the Boston Collaborative Drug Surveillance Program suggests that as many as nine percent of those who are treated with ampicillin are likely to develop a rash at some time in the two weeks following the start of treatment. This is a higher figure than earlier reports have suggested, and it is all the more serious since ampicillin is the most commonly used of the semi-synthetic penicillins. There is considerable evidence, however, that ampicillin rash is not always an allergic reaction. The evidence is provided by skin tests in which patients receive a small amount of the substance under test, just lightly pricked or injected into the skin. If the patient is truly sensitive to the substance in an allergic fashion a weal immediately arises at the point of treatment. Nearly seventy percent of people who had suffered from reactions to ampicillin have been shown not to be truly allergic to it.

There is, therefore, an unsolved problem about the nature of these adverse reactions to ampicillin. It is possible that many early cases of reaction against penicillin could have arisen from a similar unidentified mechanism. The situation is made even more complicated by the recently discovered association between ampicillin rash and mononucleosis, which is one form of what is commonly called glandular fever. No acceptable explanation of this association has yet been put forward.

In the thirty years since penicillin was developed, allergic reactions have, on the whole, been clinical problems and have been regarded as of minor importance except in those individual cases where special action is required. In very recent years, however, a new interest in penicillin allergy has arisen. In a sense this is a purely scientific interest, because it looks at penicillin allergy as a tool with which we can examine the functioning of the immune system of our bodies, rather than as a minor side-effect of a most potent drug. The research stimulated by this new interest in penicillin allergy has, however, thrown light onto a number of old clinical problems.

In principle penicillin should not be able to cause allergic reactions. The penicillin molecule is very small compared with giant macro-molecules such as the proteins which constitute much of the structure of living cells. The immune system of our bodies has evolved to protect us from attack by other organisms, and it is most effective in dealing with cells or very large molecules produced by other organisms. When working well it kills the cells of invading germs or rejects the cells of a kidney transplant. It does this by identifying the invaders as being not-self and then attacking with specially manufactured antibodies or with killer cells. It should ignore small molecules such as penicillin which are not large enough to carry the flags, or antigens, which signify that the invader is not-self. Small molecules are normally swept up by special cells (called phagocytes) whose job is clearing up debris from our systems.

It was the work of Karl Landsteiner, the man who discovered the ABO system of blood groupings, that showed that sometimes a small molecule could attach itself to a much larger molecule, a carrier, in such a way that the body would react immunologically to the combination of the two. It is certain that at least one form of penicillin allergy is brought about by a mechanism of this sort.

It has been shown experimentally that penicillin allergy can be caused by a substance called benzyl-penicilloyl-polylysine, which is usually abbreviated to BPO. The benzyl is the original side-chain of the penicillin molecule. The penicilloyl is a changed version of the penicillin nucleus after it has undergone reaction with other chemicals. The polylysine is the large carrier molecule, being made up of a number of molecules of lysine which is one of the amino-acids which are the building blocks of all proteins. It was not until 1967 that a substance of this type was discovered to be responsible for any penicillin allergy.

But the situation is not nearly so simple that it can be unraveled by a single discovery. It has been proved that BPO is not the only molecule that causes penicillin allergy. The most outstanding worker in this new field of research into penicillin allergy, Dr. Alain L. de Weck of the University of Berne in Switzerland, has shown that other breakdown products of the original penicillin molecule can certainly cause immune reactions after they have combined with protein carriers. There are cases of penicillin allergy caused by impurities in the guise of protein molecules that have been extracted from the manufacturing brew in which the drug is made and which are difficult to separate from the penicillin. There is evidence, too, that penicillin molecules can link together to form a polymer, or chain, a molecule large enough to stimulate an immune reaction but consisting only of penicillin molecules in a chain.

Further to complicate the situation it appears that these chemicals can nearly all be formed either inside the patient's body after treatment with penicillin or in the manufacturing process. BPO, for instance, can apparently be formed by at least two different chemical routes starting from the original penicillin, and each one of the necessary reactions can occur either in the body or on laboratory glassware.

The steady accumulation of knowledge about the complexity of penicillin allergy has proceeded more or less step by step in conjunction with efforts to dispose of the problem. Originally in the late 1940s it was assumed that the cause of the allergy must be impurities in the preparation of the drug, for penicillin was the product of living processes, and it was more likely that the macro-molecules of those processes would cause allergic reactions rather than the small penicillin molecule. With the arrival of the semi-synthetic penicillins it was hoped that these impurities could be removed more easily during manufacture. However, the preparation of 6-APA (the penicillin nucleus) involved treating natural penicillin G with a microbe enzyme to split off the side-chain. This, in fact, introduced yet more proteins into the preparation of the drug and increased the possibility of incorporating immunogens in the substance finally received by the patient. However, a purely chemical method of preparing 6-APA has come into use more recently that does not appear to improve the position. The introduction of a further purification stage in the manufacturing of semi-synthetic penicillins does decrease the incidence of allergic reactions to the final product. But it cannot get rid of them entirely, probably because penicillin, however pure, can react inside the body to form BPO or substances like it.

It is not possible at this time to make any useful summary of the state of knowledge about penicillin allergy; new discoveries are being made frequently. What can be said is that most people with allergic symptoms are reacting to the presence or formation of something like BPO. But there are certainly other immunogens involved in many cases, and in some cases it is these minor determinants that are alone responsible. Unfortunately, the most dangerous situation clinically—that is, the cases of anaphylactic reactions—seems to involve the minor determinants rather than BPO.

It is now known that there are at least five different sets of allergic reactions to penicillin. In addition to the anaphylactic reaction there is the "original" penicillin allergy which involves the type of antibody known as IgM. This reaction can go beyond the skin rash and angioedema that first drew attention to the problem and can escalate to fever, joint pains and even serum sickness. A rare, but different, reaction to penicillin results in the production of hemolytic anemia (a serious blood disease) in patients who have received a great deal of treatment with the antibiotic. A recently discovered fourth reaction, about which little is known, is the production of contact dermatitis when penicillin comes into frequent contact with the skin. The most recent addition to the catalog (at the time of writing) is the discovery that a small number of workers at a plant manufacturing semi-synthetic penicillins have developed asthma that has been shown to be caused by sensitivity to the inhalation of penicillin dust particles.

Chapter 17
THE FINAL TWIST

PENICILLIN and the other antibiotics act only against microorganisms, that is against bacteria, fungi and other simple creatures. But antibiotics do nothing against the other great cause of infectious disease, the viruses. And no antiviral drug of major importance has yet been discovered. (This is only a broad rule for there is one antibiotic, rifampicin, and two chemicals which seem to have clear and possibly clinically useful action against certain viruses.)

For all practical purposes it remains true that our only defense at the moment against virus diseases is protective immunization of the sort that Pasteur practiced. It is ironical that the first two vaccines developed by medicine, vaccination against smallpox and Pasteur's own rabies vaccine, gave protection against viruses which no scientist of the time could prove even to exist except by their disease-producing action.

Viruses have no cell wall for penicillin to attack, they have neither digestive nor respiratory processes for other antibiotics to interfere with. Viruses consist of nothing but genetic material (DNA or RNA) clothed in a coat of other biochemicals, usually protein. Viruses depend for their existence on the presence of living cells in the form of bacteria, other microorganisms or higher creatures such as ourselves. They enter living cells and, once there, the genetic material of the virus "takes over" the control of the machinery of the cell from the cell's own genetic material. The virus genetic material orders the cell to produce more viruses instead of getting on with its own job. More and more viruses are produced inside the cell until eventually the cell is killed and the viruses escape. For a short time the viruses are exposed to the world outside the cell, either in the body's bloodstream or even the cold atmosphere of our planet. Either they find another cell they can enter, in which case the whole process starts again, or if they are not quickly successful they are usually inactivated. There is hardly any point in this cycle where an antibiotic or other drug can attack; the viruses are usually safely hidden inside the cells we wish to protect.

It was clear to immunologists and others researching into virus diseases in the first fifty years of this century that there should be something which could at least hinder the progress of viruses in the body. It was well known that the major mechanism by which our bodies defended themselves against viruses was the production of antibodies which circulated in the bloodstream and in the lymphatic system. The antibodies neutralized and destroyed the viruses in their brief period of vulnerability when they were traveling from a killed cell to a fresh target. The production of antibodies against a virus not only cured us of disease, if the body had not died before it got a chance to manufacture enough antibodies, but also gave us immunity against further attack by the same viruses. This was the whole basis of immunization.

But in the longer term of evolution it would seem likely that the animal body had developed some protective mechanism against viruses to cover the period before the antibodies could be made in large numbers. If not, why did everyone not die at the first assault of a virulent virus? Why did some people not suffer from a particular virus disease even when they had no antibody against the virus? Why did experiments show that a very small quantity of virus injected into the body did not usually produce the appropriate disease?

In 1957 the "natural" first-line defense of the body against virus was discovered. This was not, in fact, defense by the body as a whole, as in the case of the immune system, but defense by the individual cell that was being attacked.

The man who made the discovery was Dr. Alick Isaacs, who was working in London with a young Swiss colleague, Dr. J. Lindemann. They were researching into the phenomenon known as virus interference, which appeared to be very similar to that microbial antagonism that has played such a large part in the penicillin story. It had been known for many years that the presence of one virus in a culture prevented or inhibited the growth of a second virus. (Culture in virus research means something quite different from culture in bacteriology. Because viruses will only multiply in living cells, a culture in a virology laboratory is a collection of living cells in a test-tube, or spread out in a thin layer on a glass plate.) Isaacs was investigating particularly the influenza virus and was growing the virus in hens' eggs, a process which is known technically as chick-embryo culture.

The essence of Isaacs' significant discovery was that he took a large amount of influenza viruses and killed, or inactivated, them by using mild heat or ultraviolet light so that they were no longer infectious but had not been broken up into small pieces. These inactivated viruses he injected into hens' eggs. The eggs (which consist of living cells) produced an unknown substance in response to this treatment. When this new substance was injected into further eggs, these eggs would not allow influenza virus to grow in them. The new substance was therefore an antiviral agent. It was produced by living cells in response to virus and it prevented virus growing in other living cells.

The excitement caused by Isaacs' discovery was intense. He named his new substance interferon because it interfered with virus growth. Here, it seemed to everyone, was a discovery of major importance. Not only had it been shown that cells did have a natural mechanism against virus, but also the results for medicine should prove enormously valuable. We only had to manufacture interferon by artifically stimulating cells to produce it when they did not really need it, and we could give large doses to anyone suffering from, or threatened by, a virus disease and the virus should be killed.

At first the research program into interferon went very well. It was, incidentally, supported by the N.R.D.C., determined to see that Britain did not again lose the profits that would accrue from another great discovery. Working with live viruses as well as inactivated ones it was quickly shown that interferon started to be produced by cells within a few hours of the injection of infectious material. Then it was shown that the amount of interferon steadily increased as the virus multiplied in the infected cells. Soon the multiplication of virus was stopped, apparently as the interferon did its work. Only when the numbers of virus inside the cell began to fall did the production of interferon start to fall. And the whole of this process took a few days, the time required for a normal body to start the production of large amounts of antibody.

Further research demonstrated that various different types of virus would cause cells to produce interferon. Furthermore, this interferon was the same substance whichever type of virus stimulated the cells to produce it. Next animals were treated with x-rays so as to "knock out" their immune systems and the antibody-producing mechanisms. This proved that interferon alone could enable these animals to fight off a normal infection and recover from a virus attack.

But at this stage the flow of research results slowed down. What was actually happening was that interferon was proving very difficult to handle in the laboratory, rather as penicillin had been before it, though for different reasons. One problem: only very small amounts were produced by cells. And though it was easy to disentangle interferon from the virus, because interferon would stand up to acids strong enough to disintegrate the viruses, it was remarkably difficult to separate interferon from the debris of the cell when the cell was broken up in the laboratory. It was impossible at that stage, in fact, to get pure interferon in any quantities. What little Isaacs was able to separate only served to confuse matters, because it emerged that there were either two sorts of interferon or two forms of the same interferon. All that could be said was that it was a large protein which appeared to come in two varieties that were distinguishable only by having different weights.

Even bigger snags appeared when attempts were made to develop interferon as a curative substance. It emerged that it was species-specific, e.g., mouse-cells produced mouse-interferon which could not be used in rabbits because it would cause a dangerous immune reaction, while rabbit-cells produced rabbit-interferon which could not be used in mice. So all hope of producing interferon from animals or animal-cells for use in humans had to be abandoned. (In the midst of these disappointments Alick Isaacs died, tragically young.)

Furthermore, no one could find out how interferon worked, indeed we still do not know. Our present suspicion, fifteen years after the discovery of interferon, is that interferon does not actually attack viruses; instead it seems to cause the production of another substance, not yet identified, which prevents the viruses from multiplying by denying them access to one of the vital pieces of the cell mechanism, the ribosomes. But whatever the means by which interferon deals with virus attack it is plainly something that happens inside the cell and it is difficult to see how an application of fresh or extra interferon can be injected inside a patient's cells where it can deal with the attacking virus.

Interest in interferon has only been re-aroused in the last three or four years, and mainly by the work of Maurice Hilleman and his team at the Merck Institute of Therapeutic Research at Rahway, New Jersey. They developed the approach of using an interferon inducer. The idea is to stimulate all the cells, not only those actually under virus attack, to produce more interferon. The stimulated cells will then be in a better position to resist the virus when it breaks out of the cells it has already attacked.

The essential background to the new approach is the discovery that it is only part of the invading virus that stimulates the cells to produce interferon, and the part that does this is the genetic material of the virus. In technical terms, it was discovered that double-stranded RNA was a very effective interferon inducer. But double-stranded RNA is, in fact, the genetic material of many viruses, it is like a virus without its protein coat. This, of course, explains the nature of Isaacs' original discovery; he had used inactivated influenza virus damaged by heat or ultraviolet light, and the damage was presumably (though this has not been proved) damage to the protein coat which would have revealed the genetic material inside. This, in turn, would have stimulated the egg-cells to produce interferon freely.

Hilleman's approach to the problem has been to discover a chemical which looks very like double-stranded RNA and to use this as an interferon inducer. He has found a man-made polymer, a molecule very like the long-chain molecules that make our domestic plastics, which consists of two chains twined together just like the RNA. It is called poly-IC, and it acts very well as an interferon inducer without carrying the infectious dangers of RNA.

Scientists at the Merrell Company in Cincinnati have pushed the work in a slightly different direction. They, too, have found a satisfactory interferon inducer, a substance called tilorone hydrochloride. This is a small molecule, apparently quite unlike poly-IC or RNA. This opens up the possibility of finding even further interferon inducers.

Up to the present there has been a small spate of publications in the scientific journals—from France, Britain and America—reporting results of using interferon inducers in laboratory animals. The results so far have been promising, especially in that the interferon inducers have also shown good result against tumors in animals, though whether this is the result of action by interferon is quite unknown. Some trials of interferon inducers in humans are believed to be going ahead in America.

The field is promising, though there are many distinguished people in the pharmaceutical industry who remain skeptical about interferon. This is where the final twist of the penicillin story occurs. And not surprisingly we find involved in the story no new character, but one with whom we have become very familiar: Chain.

In the mid-1960s Chain came back to England. At last he had got what he wanted, a university department equipped with a large enough pilot-scale fermentation plant. (This is the Department of Biochemistry at the Imperial College of Science and Technology in South Kensington, London. And here, as Professor Sir Ernst Boris Chain, he now rules.) But after thirty years of continuous work with the penicillium molds there was still a surprise in store for him.

It turned out that the penicillium molds could be infected, were often infected, by a virus. Indeed the virus must have been there in the penicillium molds, but quite unnoticed, throughout this story. The discovery was totally unexpected, because it had been thought that the lower molds could not be infected by viruses; they did not seem to have in themselves the conditions that viruses would find acceptable. It was known that higher fungi could be infected by viruses, and at one stage Chain called on the help of the Glasshouse Crops Research Station. This is a unit of the Agricultural Research Council, with its laboratories and experimental greenhouses at the south-coast town of Littlehampton. They are experts in the business of growing edible mushrooms for the domestic market, and they have considerable knowledge of the viruses that affect the higher fungi.

The value of this discovery of a virus in penicillium molds lay, however, not in its irony, but in the fact that the new virus was an extremely good inducer of interferon production. Basically this was because it was a very simple virus, consisting of little more than double-stranded RNA.

Further investigation showed that the most prolific carrier of the virus among the penicillia was *Penicillium stoloniferum.* The discovery of the interferon-inducing virus was again taken up by the N.R.D.C. and the first contracts for industrial research into the possibilities were taken up by Beecham Research Laboratories, continuing their cooperation with Professor Chain.

This is where the matter stands at the moment: there is much active interest, much research and some exciting preliminary results from the use of interferon inducers. But there also remains considerable skepticism and many wise and experienced pharmaceutical scientists—both in academic life and in industry—remain to be convinced of the long-term value of the approach, at least as a possible clinical weapon in medicine. Nevertheless, it remains a possibility that the penicillium molds may lead the way into the field of chemotherapy against viruses just as they did into chemotherapy against bacteria.

FINAL PERSPECTIVE

It is most unlikely that Fleming was the first scientist to see penicillin attacking germs; it is widely agreed that contamination of culture plates is a common occurrence in bacteriological laboratories. His distinction is that he was the first to be consciously aware that something of potential medical importance was happening. And he took action about what he saw.

It is equally unlikely that those patients who are recorded in the scientific and medical records as the first to be treated with, and cured by, penicillin are in fact the first to be treated and cured. For the use of molds and moldy substances for curing infections and wounds is recorded in the ancient Chinese civilizations, in the classical cultures of the Mediterranean and in west European folklore. There is even a record in historic times of a distinguished Australian scientist being offered a smelly and revolting collection of moldy material by an aborigine for his investigation, and rejecting it.

The long-term significance of penicillin may well be that it is the first example of the conscious use of a micro-organism for human purposes. The penicillium molds are the first molds to be deliberately domesticated by man. For many thousands of years men have used, and may be said to have domesticated, the yeasts which cause fermentation in the manufacture of wines and beers, and similar alcoholic drinks. But the nature of the process of fermentation, the very fact that it was caused by living, yet invisible, organisms was unknown till Pasteur unveiled the mystery in the 1860s. The deliberate cultivation and growing of fermentation micro-organisms to produce tartaric and similar acids for the food and drink industry, as practiced by Pfizer, for instance, was a direct development of the old brewing-industry techniques, based on the conscious understanding that living organisms produced the results required and that the products of their metabolism were required by man.

With the deliberate cultivation of penicillium molds to produce penicillin there is a major step forward, a change of quality, with the continued use of familiar techniques. For in the case of penicillin we have the recognition of a new type of microbial product and the deliberate selection of a strain of a micro-organism, previously unused by man, for cultivation and growth in highly artificial conditions. This qualifies the industrial manufacture of penicillin for definition as the deliberate domestication of a micro-organism.

It is now recognized by archeologists and historians that the domestication of plants and animals, which turned man from a hunter-gatherer into an agriculturalist and herdsman, was probably the most important single step in the entire history of our species. In archeology and history this step is usually called the Neolithic Revolution. Herman Kahn calls it the Agricultural Revolution to distinguish it from that other great change, the Industrial Revolution, but even under this other name it is recognized as the most important single change in man's relationship to his environment.

The Agricultural Revolution took many hundreds of years to run its course. It almost certainly took place, not once, but many times over in different parts of the world: the Middle East, India, China, Mesoamerica. In each of these separate revolutions different plants and animals were domesticated. Archeology has not yet been able to provide a precise and accurate history of how any of these revolutions occurred. But it seems consistent with the evidence to assume that the first stages in the domestication of plants and animals were not a conscious process; domestication began with the chance discovery of the mutual advantages of animals, plants and men of living together, of mutually adapting the local environment. Only later was there conscious action by man to speed the process to his advantage.

One important feature of domestication in its later stages is that it makes the animals and plants involved dependent on man and his cultivations. Modern wheat, for instance, will not survive without the field conditions man provides.

It seems that a similar process has occurred in the relationship between man and the micro-organisms. First there was the chance discovery of fermentation, with its mutual advantages to man and the yeasts. Then came the conscious step of deliberately selecting the penicillium molds and domesticating them, including the deliberate selection of particular strains of the mold and their manipulation until they have developed into strains which cannot survive without the deep-fermentation tanks that man provides.

The example of the domestication of the penicillium molds has been followed in many other fields. Micro-organisms are now used to leach out metals such as copper from piles of ore stone; many other micro-organisms have been domesticated to produce other antibiotic medicines.

Perhaps the most important, and significant, of all these domestications has been the breeding of micro-organisms to provide food from crude oil and oil products. British Petroleum, working in France and Britain, has pioneered the development of the use of microbes to produce protein from oil. A system of considerable elegance has been worked out, which uses the least wanted fraction of crude oil, the paraffin waxes, as the feed-stock. This development has already passed the pilot-plant stage and has produced enough protein for addition to animal foods on a large scale. I.C.I. has developed a different system, using different micro-organisms and different fractions of crude oil as the substrate. Shell and Amoco are moving toward industrial applications of the similar systems they have developed.

Looking further ahead, there are now proposals in the research laboratories to use genetic engineering to produce entirely new types of micro-organisms that could extract nitrogen from the atmosphere and fix it in the soil to make it available to plants at a far higher rate than any known natural micro-organisms can achieve. Experiments at the University of Sussex have successfully transferred the nitrogen-fixing genetic material—from those organisms that presently perform this function in nature—to much more common forms of bacteria. Eventually it may be possible to transfer these powers to the plants themselves, thus forming plants which provide their own fertilizer.

In the perspective of man's long history, the development of penicillin may seem more important as the first conscious domestication of a micro-organism than as the production of a drug which in its time was a "miracle."

REFERENCES
BY CHAPTER

CHAPTER 1

The quotation on page 17 comes from *Antibiotics: A Survey of Their Properties & Uses,* published by direction of the Pharmaceutical Society of Great Britain. London: The Pharmaceutical Press, 1946, p. 31.

CHAPTER 2

Although the details of the life of Pasteur can be found in any general reference encyclopedia or history of science, I have found it valuable to go back to the "official biography," published in English as *The Life of Pasteur,* by René Vallery-Radot, translated by Mrs. R.L. Devonshire. London: Constable, 1901. Other sources are:

The Birth of Penicillin by Ronald Hare. London: George Allen & Unwin, 1970. The quotation comes from page 33.

The official biography of Fleming by André Maurois, translated into English by Gerard Hopkins: *The Life of Sir Alexander Fleming,*

Discoverer of Penicillin. London: Jonathan Cape, 1959. The story of Haldane's letter to Wright can only be traced to this source.

CHAPTER 3

The Life of Sir Alexander Fleming, Discoverer of Penicillin, by André Maurois. London: Jonathan Cape, 1959; the quotation of Dr. V.D. Allison describing the discovery of lysozyme is from pp. 109, 110.

The Birth of Penicillin, by Ronald Hare. London: George Allen & Unwin, 1970; the quotation is from pp. 31 and 54.

Miracle Drug, by David Masters. London: Eyre and Spottiswoode, 1946.

An unpublished memoir on Sir Alexander Fleming by Dr. Howard Hughes, which I have also quoted.

Fleming's paper on lysozyme is *Proc. Roy. Soc.* B. 94:306.

I have also quoted from *Biographical Memoirs of Fellows of the Royal Society.* 2, 117, 1956.

CHAPTER 4

In this chapter again I am indebted to Dr. Howard Hughes, of St. Mary's Hospital Medical School (Wright-Fleming Institute) for his memoir of Sir Alexander Fleming.

The quotations are from *The Life of Sir Alexander Fleming, Discoverer of Penicillin,* by André Maurois. London: Jonathan Cape, 1959, pp. 124, 125 and 133.

Fleming's original paper is "On the antibacterial action of cultures of a penicillium with special reference to their use in the isolation of *B. influenzae.*" *British Journal of Experimental Pathology* 10:226–236.

There are also quotations from Fleming's 1946 Harben Lecture to the Royal Society of Public Health and Hygiene, *Journal of the Royal Institute of Public Health & Hygiene* 8:36.63.93. 1965, and from his speech to the American Pharmaceutical Manufacturers' Association, December 13, 1943.

CHAPTER 5

Miracle Drug, by David Masters. London: Eyre and Spottiswoode, 1946. The quotation comes from pp. 26, 27.

The Life Savers, by Ritchie Calder. London: Pan Books, 1961. The quotations come from pp. 47, 48 and 49.

Fleming, Discoverer of Penicillin by L.J. Ludovici. London: Andrew Dakers Limited, 1952. The quotation comes from p. 133.

Penicillin, A Dramatic Story, by Boris Sokoloff. London: George Allen & Unwin, 1946. Quotation from p. 20.

The Birth of Penicillin, and the disarming of microbes, by Ronald Hare. London: George Allen & Unwin, 1970. Chapters 3 and 4 describe his "detective work" and the quotations come from pp. 69 and 70.

There is also a quotation from *The Penicillin Group of Drugs,* by Gordon T. Stewart. London: Elsevier, 1965, p. 16.

I am grateful to Professor Sir Ernst Chain for permission to quote from his 1971 lecture at the Penicillin Symposium of the Royal Society and Royal College of Physicians.

The *Memoir* of Florey for the Royal Society by Professor E.P. Abraham is in volume 17 of the Society's *Memoirs,* November 1971.

CHAPTER 6

The opening quotation comes from *Antibiotics,* by H.W. Florey et al. London: Oxford, 1949.

The remainder of the chapter is largely based on *The Birth of Penicillin,* by Ronald Hare. London: George Allen & Unwin, 1970. And all the quotations come from his Chapter 5, pp. 94–102.

CHAPTER 7

The main source for this chapter is *Miracle Drug,* by David Masters. London: Eyre and Spottiswoode, 1946. Quotations from pp. 53 and 56.

Maurois and Hare both confirm details.

The Fleming quotation comes from *History and Development of Penicillin,* ed. Sir Alexander Fleming. London: Butterworth, 1946, p. 14.

CHAPTER 8

The development in the pharmaceutical industries in Britain, Europe and the U.S.A. is based upon *A History of the Modern British Chemical Industry,* by D.W.F. Hardie and J. Davidson Pratt. London: Pergamon, 1966. Quotations from pp. 76, 108 and 156.

And *The Pharmaceutical Industry,* by Wyndham Davies, M.P. London: Pergamon, 1967. Quotation from p. 1.

The arrival of the sulfa drugs, especially of Prontosil, is described by Professor Ronald Hare in *The Birth of Penicillin.* London: George Allen & Unwin, 1970, Chapter 7. All quotations come from pp. 136–144 except the final one which is from p. 161.

CHAPTER 9

Miracle Drug, by David Masters and André Maurois' *Life of Sir Alexander Fleming,* mentioned in other chapters, both give some details of previous work on bacterial antagonism.

The work of Gratia and Dath is recorded in Sokoloff's *Penicillin, A Dramatic Story.*

The papers by B. Gosio were printed in *Rivista D'Igiene e Sanita Publica, Turin* N. 21, November 1, 1896 and N. 26, December 16, 1896. I am grateful to Dr. Peter Farrago for translation.

CHAPTER 10

Miracle Drug, by David Masters. London: Eyre and Spottiswoode, 1946; and *Rise Up to Life,* by Lennard Bickel, London: Angus & Robertson, 1972, the biography of Lord Florey, have provided much background.

But I am principally grateful to Professor Sir Ernst Chain for a number of interviews in which he recalled his work for me. He also provided a manuscript of his address "Thirty Years of Penicillin Therapy" given at the Symposium on Penicillin organized by the Royal Society in London in 1971 to celebrate the thirtieth anniversary of the first successful clinical use of penicillin. This was printed in *Proc. Roy. Soc.* B. 179:293–319. All the quotations from him come from this source except for the one on pp. 159–60, which is from my interview with him.

Professor Chain also provided me with photocopies of Florey's letter to Dr. Warren Weaver of the Rockefeller Foundation and of the official application for a grant from the foundation.

Dr. N.G. Heatley, of the Sir William Dunn School of Pathology in Oxford, also allowed me to interview him and showed me his laboratory notes.

The paper "Penicillin as a chemotherapeutic agent" was published in *Lancet,* August 24, 1940, pp. 226–228.

I have also quoted from *Penicillin, A Dramatic Story*, by Boris Soko-loff. London: George Allen & Unwin, 1946, pp. 24, 25.

The quotations referring to Florey's appointment to the chair of pathology at Oxford and to his attitude to the work on penicillin come from the obituary notice in *Nature* 218:304, 305.

CHAPTER 11

Most of the material for this chapter comes from personal interviews with Professor Sir Ernst Boris Chain, Dr. Norman G. Heatley, and Professor Charles Fletcher, of the Royal Postgraduate Medical School, Hammersmith Hospital.

The Heatley quotations come from his obituary notice of Lord Florey, published as "In Memoriam, H.W. Florey: An Episode." *Journal of General Microbiology* 61:289–299.

The quotation from Chain comes from his lecture referred to in the previous chapter.

Other sources are *Miracle Drug* by David Masters and *Rise Up to Life* by Lennard Bickel.

The paper "Further observations on penicillin" was published in the *Lancet* ii:177.

The quotation from Stewart comes from *The Penicillin Group of Drugs*, by G.T. Stewart. London: Elsevier, 1965, p. 10.

CHAPTER 12

Those parts of this chapter which deal with Florey's activities are mostly based on the biography of Florey, *Rise Up to Life*, by Lennard Bickel. London: Angus & Robertson, 1972. The quotations from Florey's and Mellanby's correspondence also come from this book, pp. 135 and 136. The account of the work of Dawson, Hobby and Meyer in the U.S.A. is also based on Bickel with quotations from pp. 127–129.

The activities of Florey and Heatley in America are based on Heatley's memoir of Florey in the *Journal of General Microbiology* mentioned in Chapter 11 and all the quotations from Heatley are taken from this. Dr. Norman Heatley also provided further information in an interview with the author.

Miracle Drug by David Masters. London: Eyre and Spottiswoode, 1946. Provides most valuable information and, in particular, was written when memories of these episodes were freshest.

Florey's visit to the Connaught Institute in Toronto is described by Professor Hare in *The Birth of Penicillin*. London: George Allen & Unwin, 1970. The quotation comes from pp. 172–173.

Large-scale penicillin production in the U.S.A. was originally described by Dr. Robert Coghill and R.S. Koch in a major article, "Penicillin: a wartime accomplishment," *Chemical and Engineering News* 23: 2310–2316. This article is the basis of the section on U.S. production.

But the description of early American methods in action comes from Professor Hare, *The Birth of Penicillin*, p. 177.

The particular contribution of the Pfizer Company in America and of Kemball, Bishop in Britain is based upon information from the companies' records kindly given to me by Dr. L.M. Miall, Manager, Fermentation Development Department, Pfizer Europe Chemicals, at Sandwich in Kent, and formerly an executive of Kemball, Bishop before that company was taken over by Pfizer. Dr. Miall also gave me the benefit of his personal memories of wartime penicillin production in Britain, and he gave me access to such sources as the minutes of the General Penicillin Committee.

I am also obliged to Imperial Chemical Industries, Ltd., through Mr. Geoffrey Richards for help with details of their early work. Mr. H.W. Palmer of Glaxo allowed me a long interview and the help of his memories, especially over the problems of British industry accepting the necessity of buying deep-fermentation licenses from the U.S.A.

Masters's book *Miracle Drug* provides contemporary reporting on production of penicillin in Britain.

CHAPTER 13

The references to the London *Times* are all dated as part of the text.

The letter from Mr. Whitehall of Kemball, Bishop and the extracts from the minutes of the General Penicillin Committee have been provided from that company's records by Dr. Miall.

Some of the information contained in this chapter comes from personal interviews with Professor Sir Ernst Chain.

Professor Abraham's *Memoir of Lord Florey* has been mentioned in previous chapters. *Biographical Memoirs of Fellows of the Royal Society* 17 (November 1971).

For Florey's reactions to the press see *Rise Up to Life*, by Lennard Bickel. London: Angus & Robertson, 1972, pp. 173 and 174. And from the same source Florey's correspondence with Sir Edward Mellanby, pp. 108 and 109.

The quotation from Heatley comes from his memoir of Florey in the *Journal of General Microbiology* referred to in previous chapters.

The quotation from Fleming comes from *Miracle Drug* by David Masters, p. 118.

CHAPTER 14

The greater part of the information in this chapter is drawn by the author from his own work as a science journalist.

Interviews with Dr. B.A.J. Bard, formerly director of the National Research Development Council, provided much information.

Personal interviews were also provided by a number of officers of the Glaxo Co. Ltd.

The quotations come from that company's records in the Glaxo Volume 28.

"New Penicillins, cephalosporin C and Penicillinase," by E.P. Abraham and G.G.F. Newton. *Endeavour* XX:92–100.

CHAPTER 15

The source for the bulk of this chapter is an unpublished account of the work by Beecham Research Laboratories compiled by the former director, Dr. J. Farquharson, which Beecham has kindly allowed me to use.

Dr. Rolinson and Dr. Nayler also gave personal interviews to add their memories to the more formal account.

The quotations from Chain come from his address at the Royal Society Symposium celebrating thirty years of the clinical use of penicillin, London 1971, published in *Proc. Roy. Soc.* B. 179:293–319; and from his Frueman Wood lecture at the Royal Society of Arts June 19, 1963, reprinted in *Nature* 200:441–451.

The quotations from Professor G.T. Stewart come from *The Penicillin Group of Drugs*. London: Elsevier, 1965, pp. 34 and 35.

CHAPTER 16

I am particularly grateful to Dr. R.J. Davies of St. Thomas's Hospital and Dr. J. Amos of the Institute of Dermatology, London, for help with this chapter.

The main scientific papers referred to are: National Research Council Division of Medical Sciences Committee on Chemotherapeutic and Other Agents (1943). "Penicillin in the treatment of infections." *JAMA* 122:1217.

Jack M. Batson. "Anaphylactoid reactions to oral administration of penicillin." *New England Journal of Medicine.* 262:590–594.

A.L. de Weck. "The formation of penicillin antigens." *Proc. Roy. Soc. Med.* 61:894–897.

F.R. Batchelor, and Janet M. Dewdney. Ibid., 897–899.

Boston Collaborative Drug Surveillance Program. "Ampicillin rashes." *Arch. Dermatol.* 107 (January 1973).

C. Warren Bierman et al. "Reactions associated with ampicillin therapy." *JAMA* 220 (May 22, 1972).

R.J. Davies, D.J. Hendrick and J. Pepys. "Asthma due to inhaled chemical agents: ampicillin, benzyl-penicillin, 6-amino penicillanic acid and related substances." *Clinical Allergy* 4:233–253.

CHAPTER 17

The best summary of this current work and its origins was given by Professor Sir E.B. Chain, in his lecture to the Royal Institution in London, "Fungal viruses and their antiviral properties," given on March 3, 1972. Professor Chain has kindly given me a copy of his script.

SELECTIVE
BIBLIOGRAPHY

Bickel, Lennard. *Rise up to Life, A Biography of Howard Walter Florey Who Gave Penicillin to the World.* London: Angus and Robertson, 1972; New York: Scribner, 1973.

Calder, Ritchie. *The Life Savers.* London: Pan Books, 1961.

Davies, Wyndham. *The Pharmaceutical Industry.* London and New York: Pergamon, 1967.

Director of Medical Services, 21 Army Group, "Penicillin Therapy and Control in 21 Army Group", Her Majesty's Stationery Office, London, 1945.

Florey, H.W., Chain, E., Heatley, N.G., Jennings, M.A., Sanders, A.G., Abraham, E.P., and Florey, M.E. *Antibiotics.* London: Oxford University Press, 1946.

Goldsmith, Margaret. *The Road to Penicillin.* London: Lindsay Drummond, 1946.

Hardie, D.W.F. and Pratt, J. Davidson. *A History of the Modern British Chemical Industry.* London and New York: Pergamon, 1966.

Hare, R. *The Birth of Penicillin.* London: George Allen & Unwin, 1970.

Humphrey, J.H. and White, R.G. *Immunology for Medical Students.* Oxford: Blackwell, 1970, 3rd Edition.

Lacken, G. *The Story of Penicillin.* London: Pilot Press, 1945.

Ludovici, L.J. *Fleming, the Discoverer of Penicillin.* London: Andrew Dakers, 1952.

Masters, David. *Miracle Drug.* London: Eyre and Spottiswoode, 1946.

Maurois, André. *The Life of Sir Alexander Fleming*; translated from the French by Gerard M. Hopkins. London: Jonathan Cape, 1959; New York: E.P. Dutton, 1959.

Pharmaceutical Society of Great Britain. *Antibiotics: A Survey of their Properties and Uses.* London: Pharmaceutical Press, 1952, 3rd Edition.

Vallery-Radot, René. *The Life of Pasteur.* London: Constable, 1901; Finch Press, 1923.

Sokoloff Boris. *Penicillin, A Dramatic Story.* London: George Allen & Unwin, 1946.

Stewart, G.T. *The Penicillin Group of Drugs.* London and New York: Elsevier, 1965.

Wilson, David. *Body and Antibody.* New York: Knopf, 1972. Published in Great Britain by the Longman Group Limited, under the title *The Science of Self,* 1972.

INDEX

A NOTE ABOUT THE AUTHOR

David Wilson was born in 1927
in Rugby, Warwickshire, England. Educated at
Ampleforth College, York, and Pembroke College,
Cambridge, Mr. Wilson studied mathematics, physics, and
history, receiving a B.A. and an M.A. from Cambridge
University. A newspaper reporter from 1950 to 1955,
he joined the BBC news department in 1956, and has
been their Science Correspondent since 1963. In addition
to broadcasting regularly on BBC radio and television,
Mr. Wilson has published a number of articles in *The
Listener* and is the author of *Body and Antibody*
and *The New Archaeology*. He is married,
and the father of four children.

A NOTE ON THE TYPE

The text of this book was set by a computer and CRT
system in a type face called Baskerville. The face is a
facsimile reproduction of types cast from molds made for
John Baskerville (1706–75) from his designs. The
punches for the revived Linotype Baskerville were cut
under the supervision of the English printer George W.
Jones.

John Baskerville's original face was one of the
forerunners of the type style known as "modern face" to
printers—a "modern" of the period A.D. *1800*.

*Composed, printed and bound at
The Haddon Craftsmen, Inc., Scranton, Pennsylvania*

Designed by Gwen Townsend